HARRY'S COSMETICOLOGY 9TH EDITION

FOCUS BOOKS

Manufacturing: Process Techniques for the Cosmetic Industry

ISBN: 978-0-8206-0404-6

Harry's Cosmeticology

9th Edition

Volume One - ISBN: 978-0-8206-01762
Volume Two - ISBN: 978-0-8206-01779
Volume Three - ISBN: 978-0-8206-01786
eBook - ISBN: 978-0-8206-01793

First Edition

Chemical Publishing Company

www.chemical-publishing.com

Printed in the United States of America

A Note from the Publisher:

The new 9th edition of Harry's Cosmeticology is available as a 3 volume set containing over 2600 pages of new information on the recent changes in the cosmetic and personal care products industry.

Chemical Publishing is now offering key parts of the title for those interested in a particular subject area covered in the book.

Harry's Cosmeticology 9th Edition has developed a new line of titles called "Focus Books" for this purpose.

"Focus Books" are a series of selected chapters that can be used as a reference guide for partial subject areas covered in the parent text.

Because the chapters have been taken from the original individual volumes, the reader will find that the pages have not been renumbered in standard order starting from page one, moving forward, but rather they have been left in the original format so that the information will flow chronologically, although the pages may in fact not be numbered as so.

The benefit of leaving the page numbers as they were taken from the original text is that the reader will be able to use the Table of Contents and page numbers referenced within the Focus Book to find the desired content and we have tried to keep the chapter segments in the same order in which you would find them in the master text.

The full 3 volume Trilogy of Harry's Cosmeticology 9th Edition can be purchased through Chemical Publishing Company at www.chemical-publishing.com or through any major online retailer. It is also available in Ebook format through Kindle or as mobi, or ePub available directly from the publisher.

www.chemical-publishing.com

Our webpage featuring Authors, Reviews and other information about the 9th edition:

www.harryscosmeticology.com

About the Editor-in-Chief

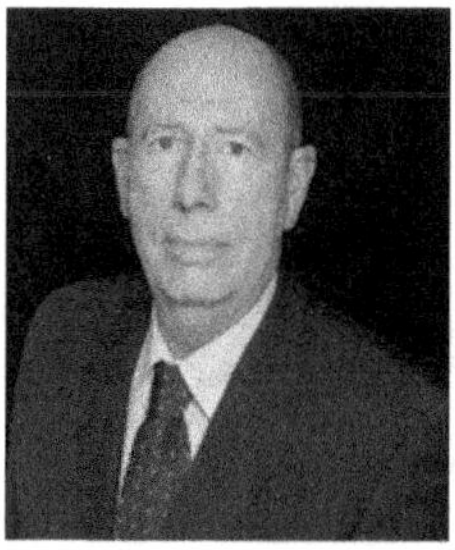

Meyer R. Rosen

CChem, CPC, CChE, CFEI, DABFE, DABFET, FAIC

Meyer R. Rosen is President of Interactive Consulting, Inc. (www.chemicalconsult.com). He is a Thought-Leader and expert in the field of Technical Marketing and multi-industry Technology Transfer Applications including, but not limited to: cosmetics and personal care, applied rheology, applied surface and interfacial chemistry, polymers, organosilicones, professional editing and custom preparation of Mind-Maps® for the organization and presentation of complex information.

Mr. Rosen is a Chartered Chemist and Fellow of the Royal Society of Chemistry (London); a Fellow of the American Institute of Chemists and both a Nationally Certified Professional Chemist and Certified Professional Chemical Engineer. He is a member of the U.S. Society of Cosmetic Chemists (SCC) & the American Institute of Chemical Engineers. Meyer serves as an Advisor for David Smith, Executive Director of the SCC Advisory Committee. He is also Editor for U.S. & Canada and Editor-in-Chief for North and Latin America for Euro Cosmetics Magazine in Germany. Mr. Rosen is Editor of the Delivery System Handbook for Personal Care and Cosmetic Products and Editor-in-Chief of Harry's Cosmeticology, 9th Ed.

Meyer served for six years as the Chief Scientific Advisor and Director of Technical Programming for United Business Media's (UBM) HBA Technical Conferences. He a former Director of the American Institute of Chemists, past Vice President of the Association of Consulting Chemists and has served on the Scientific Advisory Board of Supply Side West/East: Virgo Publications. Mr. Rosen is also the Founder, Organizer and co-moderator for HBA's Annual International Safety, Regulatory and Certification Symposia.

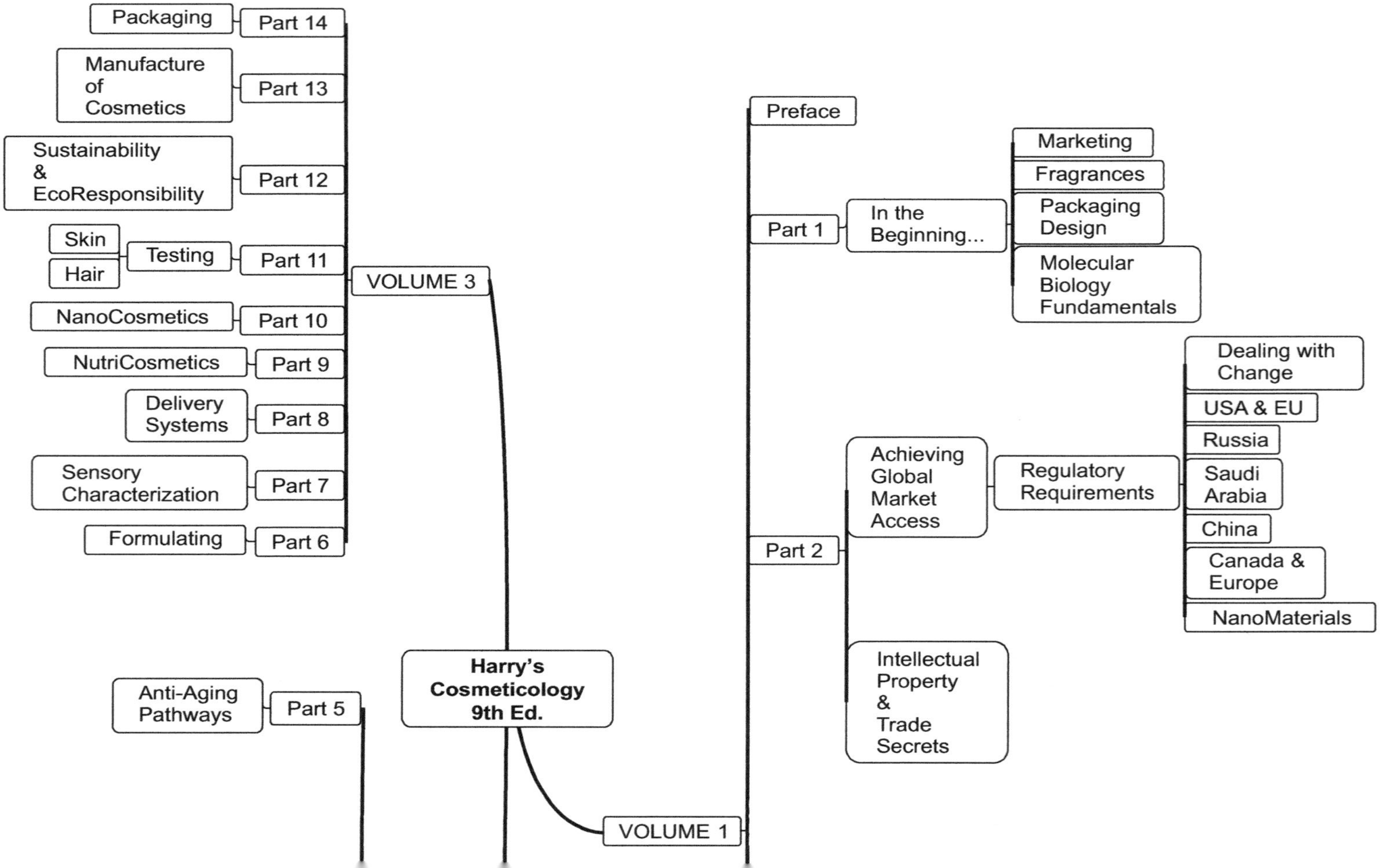

Harry's Cosmeticology 9th Ed.
VOLUME 1
Preface
Part 1
In the Beginning...
Marketing
Fragrances
Packaging Design
Molecular Biology Fundamentals
Part 2
Achieving Global Market Access
Regulatory Requirements
Dealing with Change
USA & EU
Russia
Saudi Arabia
China
Canada & Europe
NanoMaterials
Intellectual Property & Trade Secrets
VOLUME 3
Part 6
Formulating
Part 7
Sensory Characterization
Part 8
Delivery Systems
Part 9
NutriCosmetics
Part 10
NanoCosmetics
Part 11
Testing
Skin
Hair
Part 12
Sustainability & EcoResponsibility
Part 13
Manufacture of Cosmetics
Part 14
Packaging
Part 5
Anti-Aging Pathways

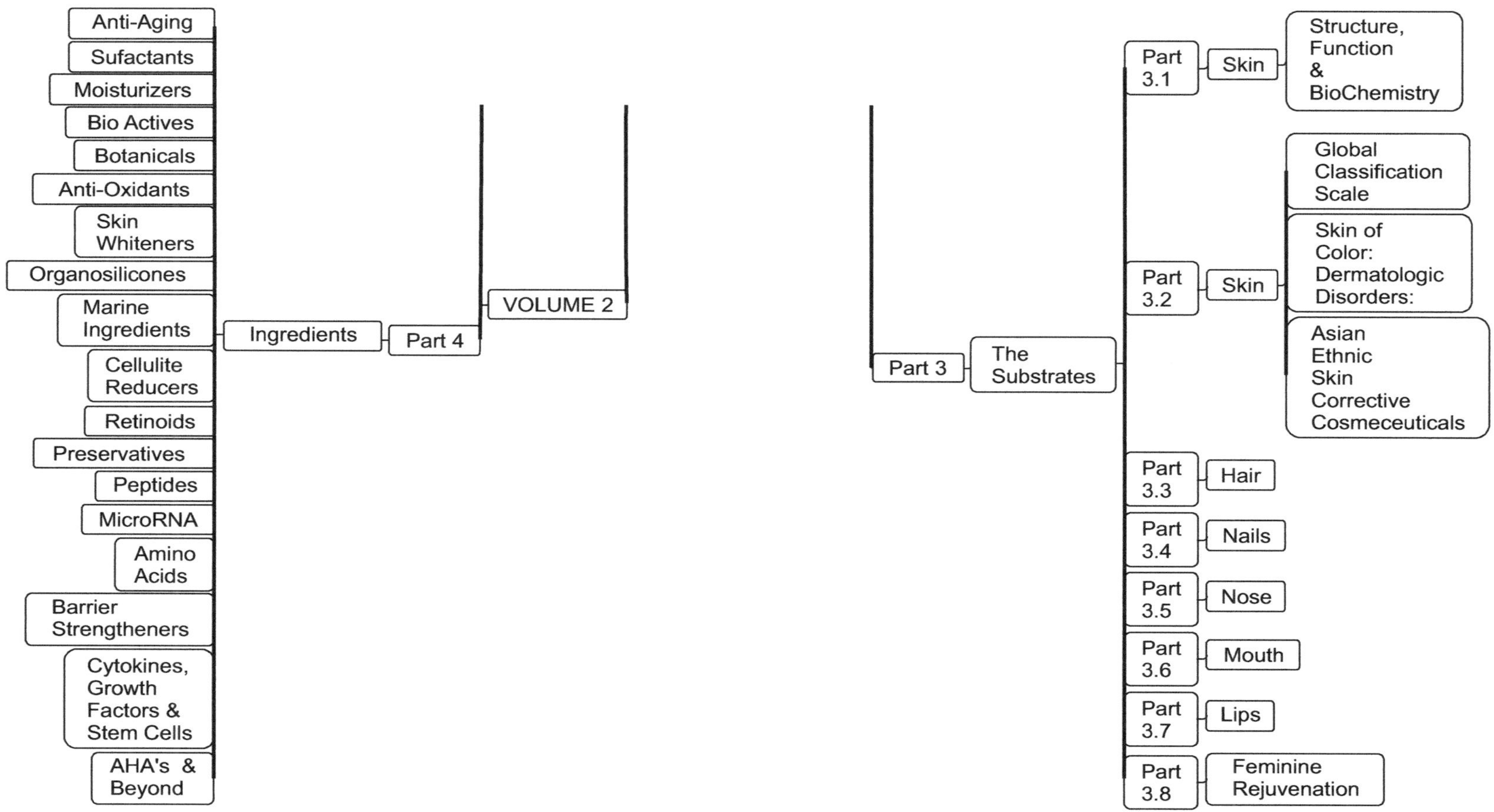
Anti-Aging
Sufactants
Moisturizers
Bio Actives
Botanicals
Anti-Oxidants
Skin Whiteners
Organosilicones
Marine Ingredients
Cellulite Reducers
Retinoids
Preservatives
Peptides
MicroRNA
Amino Acids
Barrier Strengtheners
Cytokines, Growth Factors & Stem Cells
AHA's & Beyond
Ingredients
Part 4
VOLUME 2
Part 3
The Substrates
Part 3.1
Skin
Structure, Function & BioChemistry
Part 3.2
Skin
Global Classification Scale
Skin of Color: Dermatologic Disorders:
Asian Ethnic Skin Corrective Cosmeceuticals
Part 3.3
Hair
Part 3.4
Nails
Part 3.5
Nose
Part 3.6
Mouth
Part 3.7
Lips
Part 3.8
Feminine Rejuvenation

AUTHORS

COSMETIC MANUFACTURING PROCESSES

Editor: Bruce Victor

Contributors:

Donald S. Buell

Rose Khosravani

Doug J. Melenkevitz

Bruce L. Victor

David P. Yacko

Meyer R. Rosen

COLD-PROCESS EMULSIFICATION PRODUCING

Michael Ross

James Wilmott

INTELLIGENT SELECTION AND MANUFACTURE OF NATURAL EXTRACTS

Satish Nayak

PART 13 COSMETIC MANUFACTURING

PART 13.0

MANUFACTURE OF COSMETICS SECTION OVERVIEW

PART 13.1

COSMETIC MANUFACTURING PROCESSES

Editor: Bruce Victor
Contributors:
Donald S. Buell
Rose Khosravani
Doug J. Melenkevitz
Bruce L. Victor
David P. Yacko
Meyer R. Rosen

TABLE OF CONTENTS:

PART 13.2

COLD-PROCESS EMULSIFICATION PRODUCING SUB-MICRON DISPERSIONS:
FORMULATION AND AESTHETIC ENHANCEMENT OF COSMETIC AND OTC PRODUCTS

Authors:
Michael Ross
James Wilmott
Leading Edge Innovations, LLC
50 Tannery Road, Suite #5
Branchburg, New Jersey 08876

TABLE OF CONTENTS:

PART 13.3

INTELLIGENT SELECTION AND MANUFACTURE OF NATURAL EXTRACTS

Author:
Satish Nayak, PhD
Kemin Industries,
2100 Maury Street, Des Moines, Iowa 50317, USA.

TABLE OF CONTENTS:

MANUFACTURE OF COSMETICS

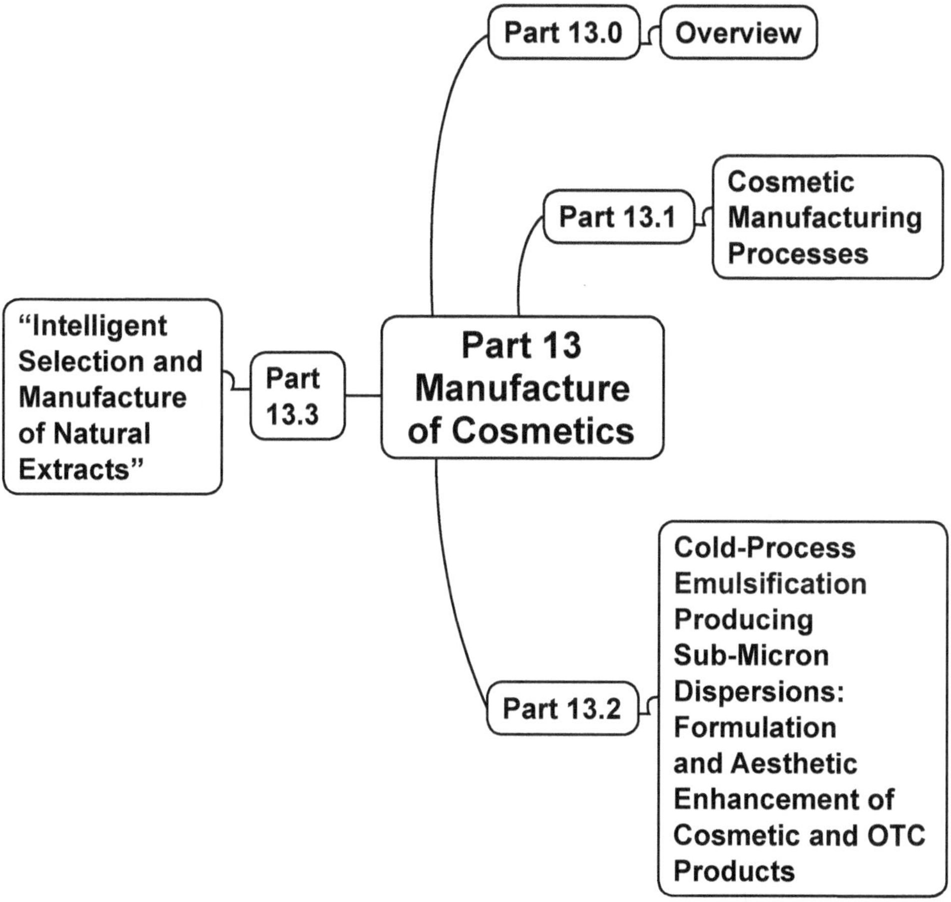

PART 13.0

MANUFACTURE OF COSMETICS SECTION OVERVIEW

As you may have noticed, this part of the book has been placed near its end. We have discussed many things in the world of cosmetics and personal care such as ingredients, anti-aging theories, and substrates including, but not limited to, skin and hair. We have delved deeply into formulating, marketing, intellectual property aspects, and global regulatory issues, to name but a few of the important areas one needs to understand as state of the art in this, the 9th Edition of *Harry's Cosmeticology*.

As we near completion of this work, we have one more major topic (besides packaging) that needs to be covered.

It is my opinion, that no matter how novel your ingredient, or its delivery system, or its formulation, sensory impact, fragrance, packaging etc., once your prototype product gets out of the lab, it must be scaled up successfully or all the work that has led to a product about to become a Brand will be for naught.

Scaling up is usually a two-step process; first to pilot scale and then to full-scale production. It is my experience that these transitions are typically fraught with angst. Some of it arises from the unfortunate fact that the ability of both laboratory developers to understand and work with individuals who are charged with making their products on a larger scale are often lacking the fine edge of successful communication. This observation, by the way, is a two-way street—for the large-scale people must also understand the laboratory people.

Even the distinction between "chemist" and "chemical engineer" creates a schism in the context described above.

To be complete in our vision to truly survey cosmetics and personal care, we must inevitably provide an understandable foundation of what the issues and approaches are when "scaling up."

To this end, we have engaged Bruce Victor and his team at Estée Lauder to provide the necessary training. Bruce is uniquely qualified for this daunting task, since he and his associates wrote the 8th Edition of *Harry's* on this subject!

Since so much has changed since the 8th Edition, you will find an enormous amount of new technology to learn about and understand. It is also my opinion that without knowing something about this area, and being able to use the information to successfully interact in the trek from concept to lab to pilot plant to full-scale production, your greatest product concept is doomed to failure.

It is with pleasure that I present the cosmetics manufacturing section by Bruce and his team. I have also taken the liberty of including two other chapters in this Part. These deal with novel emulsification and extraction technology and stand on their own, distinct from the chemical engineering, equipment, and approaches to manufacturing the many different forms of cosmetic and personal care products elsewhere in the book.

Enjoy . . .

And Learn . . .

Meyer R. Rosen

Editor-in-Chief

PART 13.1

COSMETIC MANUFACTURING PROCESSES

Editor: Bruce Victor

Contributors

Donald S. Buell
Rose Khosravani
Doug J. Melenkevitz
Bruce L. Victor
David P. Yacko
Meyer R. Rosen

ABSTRACT

Delivering the intended benefits to the consumer is the key goal for the formulating chemist. Success will help the company to grow the business. This objective is best achieved when the process used in production is controlled and reproducible. A formulator who is knowledgeable of scale-up techniques and the use of both pilot and production equipment has an advantage when the product moves out of the laboratory and into production. Armed with this knowledge, the formulator can best simulate the plant process and plan bench work effectively to ease the scale-up process and help ensure a smooth transition.

This chapter provides a brief understanding of the more important unit operations—mixing, heat transfer, and mass transfer. This is followed by a discussion of equipment, procedures, and principles commonly used in the cosmetics industry to manufacture and fill both wet and dry products. Also included is a brief discussion on drug (active) delivery systems and their special formulation/process requirements and interactions. This leads to the concept of formulations based upon the process instead of a process designed to handle the formulation. The sections on scale-up of both wet and dry products are particularly important since product quality and stability may be adversely affected as the process progresses from bench to production. For this reason it is recommended that the formulator plan the use of bench equipment and procedures carefully with pilot and full-scale limitations in mind.

This background, combined with time spent in both the pilot and manufacturing plants, will better equip the formulator to carry out successful new product introductions.

TABLE OF CONTENTS

13.1 INTRODUCTION

This chapter begins by providing a brief understanding of the more important unit operations, namely mixing, heat transfer, and mass transfer. This is followed by a treatment of equipment, procedures, and principles commonly used in the cosmetics industry to manufacture and fill both wet and dry products, including some newer approaches to the emulsion system concepts. Knowledge of this background, combined with time spent in both the pilot and manufacturing plants, will equip the effective formulator to carry out successful new product introductions.

The sections on scale-up of both wet and dry products are particularly important since cosmetic and personal care product quality and stability may be adversely affected as the process progresses from bench to production. For this reason it is recommended that the formulator plan the use of bench equipment and procedures carefully with pilot and full-scale limitations in mind. We highly recommend formulators to generate a purposeful coordination and communication with pilot plant and full-scale manufacturing experts in order to achieve a mutual understanding that each approach, from bench to full-scale, has its own inevitable strengths and weaknesses and it is only through excellent communication that successful production will be achieved.

Formulating cosmetic and personal care products is an ancient art. Originally, these products contained ground minerals in an oil or grease. They were initially used by men to exaggerate their features during battle, to conduct tribal ceremonies, and to differentiate different tribes or clans. The use of cosmetics by women began in ancient Egypt. Color products accentuated facial features; plant and animal essences provided a scent to the hair and body (minimizing body odor); and greases and oils were used to treat the skin. Skin care did not really change over the years and typically involved the application of natural oils or glycerin and rosewater preparations.

A Brief Chronological Survey

The first widely used cosmetic dates back to AD 200 when the Greek physician, Galen, published a formula that contained only rose water, beeswax, and olive oil. This formula remained essentially unchanged until the late 1800s, when borax was added to the basic formula to form a simple cold cream preparation. The principal cleansing agent at the time was a lye-based soap made by mixing potash or lye with animal or vegetable-based fats. The art of soap-making became more refined throughout the second millennium.

The era of modern cosmetics emerged in the 1940s with the widespread use of synthetic surface-active agents. These materials, commonly called surfactants, modified the surface tension of the oil and water phases and enabled the formulator to mix them together to form a composition that was stable for at least the commercial shelf life of the product. These preparations were called emulsions and the surface-active materials used to form them were called emulsifiers. Personal care products continued to evolve throughout the latter part of the 20th century. Raw material manufacturers improved aesthetic sensations through the use of new, more refined natural oils and synthetic emollients, thereby allowing product forms to become more diverse. Traditionally skin care products were moisturizers. They were used to treat dry skin by plasticizing and softening the hard, rough, tight, scaly manifestations of damaged skin.

In the late 1960s and early 1970s functional skin treatment products emerged. Product performance expanded beyond the amelioration of superficial dryness, and benefits evolved to a higher therapeutic level. The boundary between cosmetics and dermatological drug products began to blur. Problems such as aging, uneven skin pigmentation, slack skin, cellulite, sensitive skin, oily skin, and dryness were identified and agents were sourced, or developed, to address these conditions—most as cosmetics, some as dermatological (drug) products. These skin disorders were often associated with conditions such as sunburn, acne, or the need for topical analgesia, etc. The personal care market started to borrow from the latest advances in medical research. Processing these new formulations has become even more important to maintain the required aesthetics and stability required by the consumer.

In the 40 years since the late 1970s, formal chemical engineering concepts began to be introduced into the manufacture of cosmetics and personal care products. There appeared a schism between formulators (chemists) and process engineers (usually chemical engineers). Their scholastic training overlapped, but communication within an organization was often far from perfect. Yet, while these disciplines can be very diverse, the successful development of commercial cosmetics requires a smooth transition from bench to pilot to full-scale production.

Within the recent past, OTC (over-the-counter drugs) protocols have added multiple layers of regulations and paperwork to be handled from both R&D and Production. Anti-dandruff shampoos, antiperspirants, and sunscreen products are much more common. Also included in these changing times is the emphasis on "organic" and "natural"—two words that indicate potential issues related to raw materials (consistency), formulation (control of aesthetics), and process (control of the uncontrolled).

In this chapter, we focus primarily on the chemical engineering principles without which pilot and full-scale manufacture would be nonexistent. In the spirit of *Harry's* long history of explaining concepts in simple terms, we have taken the approach of examining the areas most important to gaining a true understanding of what it takes, at the full-scale production end of the process, to generate mass-scale production of products creatively generated in the laboratory—both through the creative thinking of "ingredient-seekers" to formulators to (and from) marketers. We seek to acknowledge all of the people who contribute to making new products and brands successful.

We begin with Unit Operations, the heart of understanding the basics of full-scale production.

13.1.2 UNIT OPERATIONS

When studying scale-up operations, wherever they originate, and no matter how complex, one considers a limited number of physical phenomena. These are separated into discrete yet interdependent events called "unit operations." The manufacture of cosmetics can be described in terms of four operations:

- Fluid Flow / Mixing
- Heat Transfer
- Mass Transfer and
- Filtration

All phases of cosmetic manufacture involve aspects of each.

Fluid Flow attempts to define operations involving movement of fluids and solids exhibiting fluid-like behavior. Mixing and agitation, pumping, and metering of liquids are typical operations studied in fluid flow.

Heat Transfer involves the movement of thermal energy in a gradient from areas of higher temperature to areas of lower temperature. Heating and cooling of cosmetic bulk by conduction, convection, and radiation are studied.

Mass Transfer operations define phenomena that involve movement of components of a mixture in a concentration gradient from areas where the concentration of a component is high to areas where it is lower. Cosmetic processes can make use of mass transfer by absorption (e.g., addition of binder to a cosmetic powder) and diffusion (e.g., migration of an active ingredient). The formation of an emulsion itself can be described in terms of mass transfer.

Filtration is not usually a unit operation of major importance in cosmetics manufacture except in the production of spirituous preparations (astringents/toners, colognes, aftershaves, and perfumes). It is possible to regard filtering as unmixing, and certainly the flow characteristics of the filtered product are again of prime importance. Filtration is usually included in the process to ensure clarity. The use of sub-micron filters for the sterilization of water is discussed elsewhere in this chapter.

Each of these four unit operations involves mathematical treatments that are, perhaps, inappropriate for this book and not pertinent to our practical use of the operations. Their theoretical treatment can be found in any good chemical engineering textbook, such as *Unit Operations of Chemical Engineering* by Mc-Cabe and Smith.

Mixing and heat transfer are the most critical operations and will be discussed in some detail [1].

a. Mixing

The subject of bulk cosmetics manufacture revolves around satisfactory mixing. There are several types of mixing employed as indicated in Table 13.1 below.

Table 13.1: Scope of mixing operations within the cosmetics industry

Type of mixing	Examples
Gas/Liquid (a) Cohesive (b) Segregative	(i) Dispersion (aeration and gasification) (i) Deaeration or degassing
2. Liquid/Liquid (A) Miscible (a) Cohesive (b) Distributive (B) Immiscible (a) Cohesive (b) Distributive (c) Segregative	(i) Chemical reactions (formation of salts from acid and base) (ii) Blending (spirituous preparations, clear lip gloss products) (iii) Pumping (low-viscosity system) (i) Blending (flow controlled) (ii) pH control or soap formation from fatty acid and base (iii) Pumping (high-viscosity system) (i) Emulsion formation (dispersion–addition rate is not critical) (i) Emulsion formation (dispersion–addition rate is critical) (i) Coalescing / Settling (phase separation)
3. Solid/Liquid and Liquid/Solid (a) Cohesive (b) Distributive (c) Segregative	(i) Dissolution (of water-soluble dyes, preservatives, powder surfactants, etc.) (ii) Suspensions and dispersions (mascara, pigments in castor oil and in other liquids) (iii) Hot pour products (lipsticks, etc.) (i) Controlled addition of liquid binders or actives to powders (i) Filtration, sedimentation, decantation
4. Solid/Solid (a) Segregative (b) Cohesive	(i) Free flowing powders discharged from hoppers, etc. (i) Face powders, eye shadows, and all dry mixing

Types of mixing:

Cohesive mixing - natural or forced combining of particles during blending
Segregative mixing - natural or forced separation of particles during blending
Distributive mixing - controlled or uniform diffusion of particles during blending

Table 13.1 represents a convenient way of classifying the mixing processes most commonly found within the cosmetics industry. Almost every cosmetic manufacturing process includes at least one mixing operation and often more than one type is involved. For example, the manufacture of a pigmented emulsion-based foundation cream may include:

(i) Preliminary dry blending of pigments and excipient (type 4b- i).
(ii) Dissolution of oil-soluble and water-soluble materials separately in their appropriate phase (type 3a- i and type 2Aa- ii).
(iii) Dispersion or suspension of pigments in the oil or water phase (type 3a- ii).
(iv) Mixing of the two phases to form an emulsion, possibly with the formation in situ of soap as part of the emulsifier (types 2Ba and 2Bb).
(v) Adjustment of pH (type 2Ab- ii).
(vi) Deaeration of the bulk (type 1b- i).
(vii) Shade matching (type 3a- i or -ii and iii).
(viii) Pumping into a storage vessel (type 2Ab- iii).

Not only are all these operations different from each other, but at each stage the characteristics of the bulk are quite different and require a different set of processing characteristics to achieve an optimal economic process. Not surprisingly, the optimum is rarely achieved throughout the process.

The subject of **pumping** is not clearly separated from that of **mixing** since the pumping process implies the forced flow of product. Any flow will naturally introduce an element of mixing if the product is not already homogeneous. Further, since flow is a common element of both processes, the same product characteristics (e.g., rheological behavior) must be taken into account in each process. Different types of pumps provide different quantities of shear to the product and thus provide different degrees of mixing. The "standard" in the industry is the positive displacement pump, which imparts little shear and thus little mixing to the product. The centrifugal pump works similarly to a propeller mixer in a frame. This pump can impart a great deal of shear and produce vigorous mixing. It is typically used with lower-viscosity materials.

1. Quality of Mixing

Mixing can only occur by relative movement between the particles of the constituent components. Three basic mechanisms for achieving this relative movement are bulk flow, convective mixing, and diffusive mixing.

- **Bulk flow** (which includes shear mixing, cutting, folding, and tumbling) occurs in pastes and solids when relatively large volumes of mixture are first separated and then redistributed to another part of the mixing vessel.
- **Convective mixing** involves the establishment of circulation patterns within the mixture (e.g., propeller mixing).
- **Diffusive mixing** occurs by particle collisions (e.g., thermal diffusion and concentration diffusion). In miscible liquids of sufficiently low viscosity, the thermal energy of the constituent molecules may be enough to achieve a good mixing by thermal diffusion without additional energy.

It is incorrect to assume, however, that the relative movement between mixture particles brought about by these mechanisms always results in an improved mixture quality or homogeneity. Many mixing problems arise from the tendency of mixture particles to segregate or aggregate during attempts to mix them, particularly with powders.

Segregation is defined as the preference of the particles of one component to be located nonrandomly in one or more sites in a mixture. The size of the nonuniformities in an imperfect mixture is sometimes referred to as the "scale of segregation" and the difference in composition between neighboring volumes is the "intensity of segregation." Segregation is fortunately not a major problem in cosmetics manufacture although it does manifest itself occasionally (e.g., the flotation of pigments during lipstick processing).

Aggregation is defined as the preference for the particles of one component to join with another component or components and then travel through the batch as a group. The aggregation can be physical (mixing of different-viscosity materials), physical bonding (powder agglomerations), or Van der Waals attractive forces leading to agglomeration of an emulsified droplet forming a loosely bound cluster of many individual droplets that may be shear sensitive and therefore produce smaller clusters at higher shear rates and pseudoplastic rheological behavior (i.e., viscosity decreases with increasing shear rate). To best control the distribution of some raw materials, aggregation may be required; cohesive powders may be included in the formula or the process may be used to develop an aggregation that is easily controlled. Surfactant/emulsifier selection and concentration can control the degree of agglomeration and final product stability/behavior.

Some products can be made without heating but these systems preclude the use of higher melting-point materials that can add richness to the aesthetics of the final product. Further, if the rate of mixing is high, there is a chance that air can be entrapped in the emulsion. This phenomenon causes an undesirable decrease in the specific gravity of the product and an artificial increase in product viscosity. Any variability in processing can lead to a range of undesirable rheological and textural properties. This issue can occur even if the formulation is not modified.

The term **"product by process"** is well known in the patent art and describes the above-stated phenomenon. If two or more formulators prepare the same product, the resulting compositions may vary considerably. This variation can occur even though each person utilized the same lots of raw ingredients. This occurs because it may be very difficult to exactly reproduce all of the processing parameters used to make an emulsion, for example. If any of the processing variables are modified unexpectedly, particle size variations may occur, or the crystalline properties of the emulsion can be compromised. Table 13.2 is a chart containing the results from an experiment to determine the effect of processing on the final properties of a 5% petrolatum-containing cream. All preparations contained the same lots of ingredients. The data demonstrate that the viscosity and specific gravity can vary dramatically depending upon the processing parameters employed to make the batch.

Table 13.2: Petrolatum Cream (5%) - Standard Emulsion Test Results

Sample 1: Optimum manufacturing procedure				
Sample 2: Overheated phases				
Sample 3: Forced cooling				
Sample 4: Ambient cooling				
Sample 5: Paddle mixing				
Sample 6: Rapid homogenization				
Sample 7: Under heated phases				
Sample	*Specific Gravity*	*Initial Viscosity (cP)*	*Viscosity (cP) 24 Hr @ 25°C*	*Viscosity (cP) 24 Hr. @ 50°C*
1	0.912	99,970	140,580	26,560
2	0.937	85,910	93,720	29,690
3	0.952	93,720	109,340	29,700
4	0.941	51,550	96,840	131,200
5	0.959	62,480	85,910	78,100
6	0.803	112,460	124,960	20,620
7	0.931	51,550	96,840	20,600
Note: Viscosity measurements were taken with a Brookfield LVT model viscometer				

There is foreseeable uncertainty at the "bench" level in the laboratory that a typical 500-gram to 2000-gram laboratory preparation will translate well to a manufacturing environment. This concern is often well founded. To deal with the vagaries of scale-up, the product may be subjected to a wide range of processing variations in order to optimize the conditions of manufacture. Products made at each level of scale-up are typically subjected to accelerated stability testing in order to ensure the integrity of the product for its anticipated shelf life. A significant alteration to the past "tried-and-true" systems or the development of an entirely new system is often laced with unknown issues that can severely jeopardize the introduction (timing) of a new product.

2. *Mixing Rheology*

Apart from the "dry" powder processing discussed later, the processes listed in Table 13.1 involve mostly liquids present in sufficiently large quantities as to impose fluid characteristics on the mixture. Although there are similarities between the flow of powders and the flow of liquids, it is easier to set up and sustain flow patterns in liquids. This makes liquid mixing processes easier to perform with a much larger variety of equipment from which to choose.

However, even for liquids the science of mixing has not yet been sufficiently developed to enable the optimal mixer to be designed for a given process from purely theoretical calculations. Much of the knowledge we have is empirical and has been accumulated from trial-and-error practical experience. Application of Computational Fluid Dynamics (CFD, a method of mathematically modeling moving systems) promises to enhance the theoretical understanding of how forces are transmitted through a fluid by a given mixer design. The use of **tomography** in specially designed laboratory and pilot systems (glass or clear plastic vessels) have provided actual measurements that can be used to verify CFD results and designs. Most of these are specialized, controlled systems using plastic beads or liquid latex spheres moving through a water or a glycol system. The liquid makes the movement easy to see and measure using lasers. Several agitation blades have been developed, modified, and improved since the 1990s using this technology. CFD now allows the models to be developed using computers alone. 3D printers can then be used to create the test pieces to confirm the designs.

By definition, fluid mixing occurs when an applied force (e.g., a moving mixer blade) creates a velocity gradient, also known as the rate of shear, in the fluid. The "layers" or "particles" that make up the fluid are moving at different velocities relative to each other while the mixing blade is exerting the force. On the other hand, agitation occurs when the fluid particles and blade are moving at the same velocity, much like droplets of cream swirling around in a cup of coffee. In the coffee and cream example, mixing does not occur until blade speed is increased sufficiently to create a velocity gradient that breaks up the cream droplets into a fine dispersion that we know as "café-au-lait."

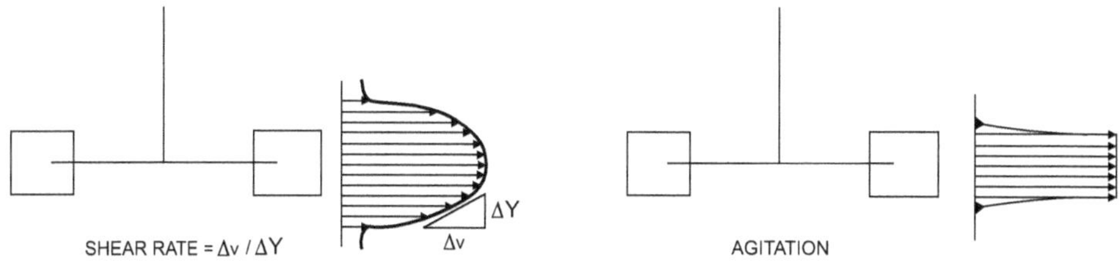

Figure 13.1: Shear rate and agitation profiles [2]

Not only is there a great variation in the physical form and properties of substances that the cosmetics industry needs to mix, but there is also a divergence of purpose. As indicated by Table 13.1, it is convenient to consider two cases separately; the first, in which the liquid components are all mutually soluble (miscible liquids), and the second, in which some or all of them can coexist as separate phases (immiscible liquids, at best partly soluble in each other).

Some mixing operations involve simple blending of miscible ingredients, for example the blending of color solutions into miscible liquids and the blending of oils, alcohol, and water in perfumes and colognes. Mixing of miscible liquids represents the simplest mixing operation in cosmetics manufacture and is achieved by developing bulk flow throughout the vessel. On the other hand, the formation of an emulsion from two immiscible phases, the suspending of a gelling agent, and the distribution of pigment agglomerates in a viscous liquid all require hydraulic shearing to break up the constituents of the mixture into finer particles during the mixing process. For this reason, such mixing is referred to as **high-shear mixing** in order to distinguish it from **simple blending**.

On the industrial scale, mixing occurs as the result of forced bulk flow within the mixing vessel. Two types of flow can be distinguished—laminar and turbulent.

Laminar flow occurs when the fluid particles move along streamlines parallel to the direction of flow. The only mode of mass transfer is by molecular diffusion between adjacent layers of fluid (Brownian motion). Heat transfer is accomplished by the same type of mechanism—conduction from layer to layer.

In **turbulent flow**, the fluid elements move not only in parallel paths but also on erratic and random paths, thus producing eddies which transfer mass from one layer to another. For this reason, turbulent mixing is rapid compared with other mixing mechanisms. Heat transfer is also influenced by forced convection—moving heat from higher- to lower-temperature areas along eddies created by turbulent mixing.

When a liquid at rest is slowly stirred the flow is laminar, but as the liquid's velocity increases flow will eventually become turbulent. A valuable aid in describing the critical point at which laminar flow becomes turbulent is due to Osborne Reynolds who, in 1883, first characterized turbulence. The dimensionless number that bears his name, N_{Re}, can be calculated for an impeller mixing in a tank as follows:

$$N_{Re} = \frac{C\,D^2 N \rho}{\eta}$$

Where N_{re} = Reynolds Number In Dimensionless Units

D = Diameter Of The Impeller In Centimeters

N = Impeller Speed In Revolutions Per Minute

ρ = Density Of Liquid In Grams Per Cubic Centimeter

η = Viscosity Of Liquid In Centipoise

C = Conversion Constant Of 1.67×10^{-4}

Equation 13.1 Reynolds Number

Experience has shown that the onset of turbulence occurs at Reynolds Numbers above 2,000. For fully developed turbulence, Reynolds Numbers greater than 10,000 are required and these higher values are found in many cosmetic mixing processes. As shown in Equation 13.1, it becomes more difficult to achieve turbulence as the viscosity (η) increases. Between 1000 and 10,000 centipoise, the viscosity range of many cosmetic products, turbulent flow can be achieved without the need for an excessive amount of power. For highly viscous creams and pastes, mixing raises certain problems since the flow pattern in the mixer is invariably laminar. Under these circumstances, distributive mixing (cutting and folding) is more applicable than turbulent mixing. Turbulence not only provides rapid mixing but also influences dispersion (mass transfer) and heating/cooling (heat transfer).

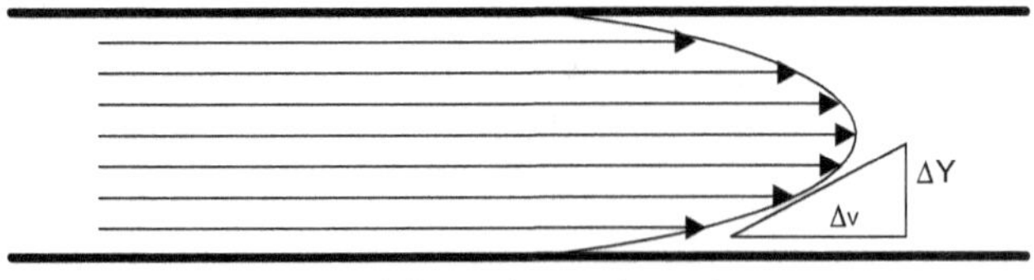

Figure 13.2: Velocity gradient of flow through a pipe

As can be seen by examining flow through a pipe Figure 13.2, there is a velocity gradient between the layers of moving liquid. A similar gradient can be found with the movement of all materials. When Newtonian (or ideal) liquids flow, the relationship between the force causing the movement (F) and the velocity gradient (ν) between the layers of moving liquid is as follows:

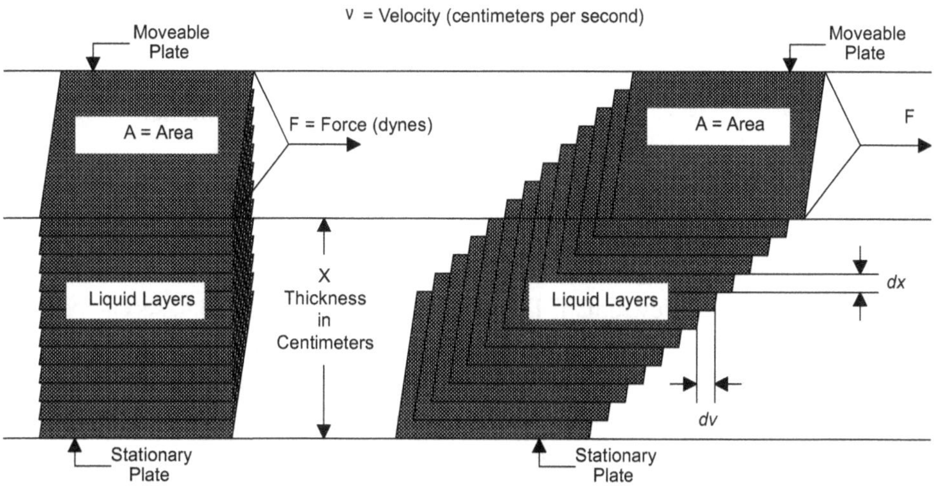

Figure 13.3: Newtonian flow [3]

F/A is commonly referred to as the "shear stress" and the velocity gradient (ν) as the "rate of shear." Assuming an ideal fluid, as velocity of flow increases, so does shear stress. This is the force that breaks up the weak bonds holding together pigment aggregates or other immiscible phases into droplets. Shear forces are also produced when liquids flow under laminar conditions, but under these circumstances the energy used to generate flow is dissipated largely as heat. During turbulent flow, the energy is dissipated in disorder; eddies are produced whose size and intensity depend upon the viscosity of the liquid and upon the force F. For a liquid of a given viscosity, the droplet size of an emulsion or the fragmented size of dispersed pigment agglomerates depends primarily on the energy input from the agitator, the velocity gradient, and the nature of the forces holding together the disintegrating entities. Unfortunately, the simple model shown in Equation 13.2 has limited application in cosmetics manufacture.

$$F = \eta \times A \times \nu$$

Where F = Force in gram-centimeters per second squared

η = Coefficient of Viscosity of Liquid in gram per centimeter-second squared

A = Cross-sectional Area of the liquid in square centimeters

ν = Velocity Gradient in centimeters per second

Equation 13.2 Force relationship to viscosity

The majority of products exhibit non-ideal (non-Newtonian) behavior, which can often be more appropriately described by the Equation 13.3.

$$F = (\eta_{app})^{n} \times A \times \nu$$

Where: F = Force in gram-centimeters per second squared

η_{app} = Apparent Viscosity of Liquid in gram per centimeter-second squared

n = exponent

A = Cross-sectional Area of the liquid in square centimeters

ν = Velocity Gradient in centimeters per second

Equation 13.3 Force relationship to apparent viscosity

In the case where the exponent, n, has a value between 0 and 1, the type of behavior is "pseudoplastic." The basic difference between materials exhibiting this property and ideal or "Newtonian" fluids is illustrated in Figure 13.4. As can be seen, pseudo plasticity is manifested by a decrease in viscosity with increasing shear rate at constant temperature. Many cosmetic liquids exhibit this behavior, especially emulsions and suspensions of particles 1 μm or less in size. Pseudoplastic viscosity loss is usually reversible; since apparent viscosity decreases as the shear rate increases and then increases along the same path as the shear rate is decreased; thus, when left unstirred long enough, the fluid will recover some or most of its original viscosity. The magnitude of the pseudoplastic effect is variable with the identity of the fluid, although a fall in viscosity of 25% when the rate of shear is doubled is not unusual.

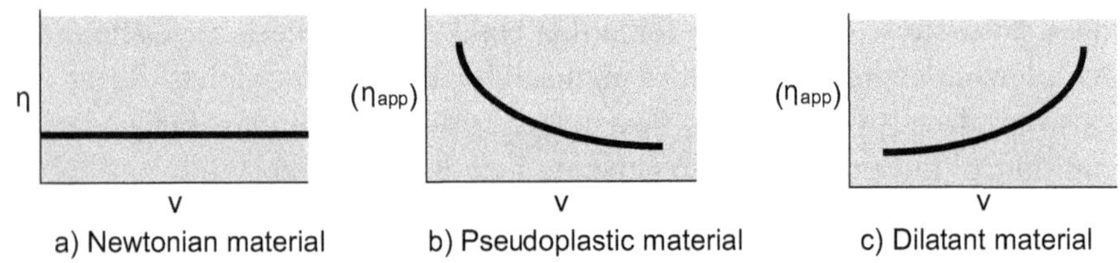

Figure 13.4 Rate of shear (ν) plotted against viscosity (η) or apparent viscosity (η_{app})

Three other types of rheological behavior are also worth noting, although they are less frequently encountered in cosmetics processing. A truly "plastic" fluid exhibits viscosity versus shear rate curves similar to those of pseudoplastic materials, but a certain force must be applied before any shear (or flow) takes place. "Dilatant" materials show the opposite effect, viscosity increasing with shear rate, Figure 13.4 c. The term "thixotropic" is often used erroneously to describe pseudoplastic behavior. Thixotropic liquids exhibit a decrease of viscosity with time at constant shear rate, not with increasing shear rate as Figure 13.4 b shows for a pseudoplastic material. However, like the pseudoplastic material, the thixotropic liquid usually recovers most of its original viscosity after the mixing force is removed. An excellent overview of the various rheological behaviors and both their mathematical characterization by empirical constants as well as their useful graphical characterization can be found in Part 1 of the *Rheology Modifiers Handbook* by David B. Braun and Meyer R. Rosen, 1999, William Andrew Publishing/ Elsevier Publishing. The authors, well familiar with the discomfiture of mathematics in the chemist's realm have provided graphical representations of the various equations and pointed out the value of what they term "Practical Rheology," where the empirical constants in the many equations can be usefully related to performance parameters of cosmetic and personal care products.

In the mixing of fluids, all three mixing mechanisms—bulk flow, turbulent diffusion, and molecular diffusion—are usually present. As viscosity increases, however, and turbulence becomes more difficult to establish, the parts played by turbulent and molecular diffusion become less important. Mixing equipment can be divided into two categories, depending on whether or not turbulent conditions prevail, as follows:

Table 13.3: Types of mixing equipment

Laminar Shear / Distributive Mixers	**Turbulent Mixers**
Helical Screw / Ribbon Blenders	Turbine-Agitated Vessels
Two-Blade Mixers	Pipes
Kneaders	Jet Mixers
Extrusion Devices	Sparged Systems
Colanders	High-Speed Shear Mixers
Static Mixers: Low N_{Re}	Static Mixers: High N_{Re}
Contra-Rotational and Planetary Side-Wiping Blades at Low Speed	Contra-Rotational and Planetary Side-Wiping Blades at High Speed

Control of mixing parameters and of the rheological characteristics of the bulk allows the manufacture of products with optimum homogeneity and stability. Heat and mass transfer are functions of the mixing process. The same mixing parameters that achieve ingredient homogeneity also influence heat and mass transfer. Good heat-transfer and good mass-transfer are both consequences of good mixing.

3. *Heat Transfer*

The topic of heat transfer in cosmetic operations does not require mathematical treatment as much as methodologies for its use and control in processing and scale-up. Heat can be used to one's advantage in a formulation. One must be aware of the fact that what can be done on the laboratory bench may not be achievable in production. The process team must be aware of the capabilities of available production-sized kettles and of the amount of heating and cooling capacity available to them.

The manufacture of most cosmetic creams and lotions involves the formation of an emulsion in which an oil and/or wax phase is combined with a water phase. This combination is made most often at higher temperatures. The even distribution of temperature is of major importance in the formation of a good emulsion. Control of the rates of heating and cooling is required in order to scale properly from bench to production and if the formulation is to be reproducible from batch to batch.

The relationship of heat and mass transfer to mixing is similar and can be treated as analogous phenomena. The degree of heat transfer depends upon a relative temperature difference (temperature gradient), which provides the driving force toward equilibrium. Equilibrium means that the temperature difference between transfer medium and product is zero. In reality, the maintenance of a gradient is required to meet the desired endpoint in heating or cooling the product, namely the "set point temperature." At this temperature we want to stop the heating or cooling process, and this is done by making the gradient zero.

The mathematical relationship between heat transferred (Q) and temperature gradient (ΔT_{LM}) is expressed below.

$$Q = U_o A_o \Delta T_{LM}$$

Where: Q = Heat transfer in watts

U_o = Overall heat transfer coefficient in watts per square meter °C

A_o = Heat transfer area in square meters

ΔT_{LM} = Log Mean Temperature gradient between the product and the heat transfer fluid (difference) in °C

Equation 13.4 Heat transfer

ΔT_{LM} takes into account the multiple heat transfer losses in the process system. The amount of heat transferred is directly proportional to the size of the temperature gradient, the contact area between heat transfer surfaces, and the magnitude of the heat transfer coefficient.

U_o is composed of a number of factors and is expressed as follows:

Where: U_o = Overall heat transfer coefficient in watts per square meter °C

H_c = Individual heat transfer coefficient between the process fluid (the product) and surface—based on the area and Δt (temperature gradient) between the surface and the fluid—in watts per square meter °C

H_{dC} = Individual heat transfer coefficient between the process fluid and surface— when that surface is fouled—in watts per square meter °C

X_w = Thickness of vessel wall in meters

K_w = Thermal conductivity of vessel wall in watts per meter °C

H_{dH} = Individual heat transfer coefficient between the heat transfer fluid (steam or cold water) and surface—when that surface is fouled by scale—in watts per square meter °C

H_H = Individual heat transfer coefficient between the heat transfer fluid (steam or cold water) and surface—based on the area and Δt (temperature gradient) between the surface and the fluid—in watts per square meter °C

Equation 13.5 Heat transfer coefficient

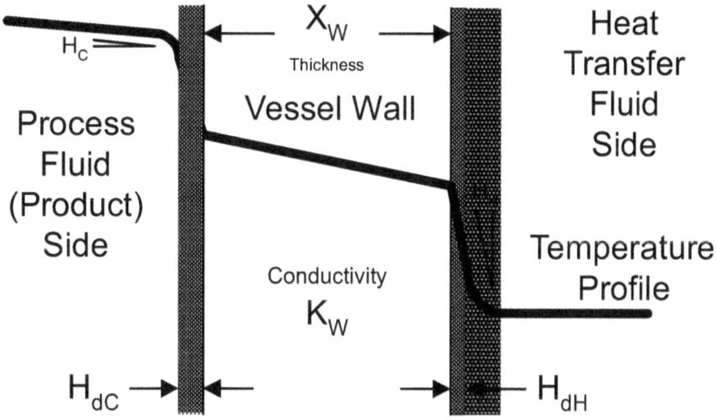

$$\frac{1}{U_O} = \frac{1}{H_C} + \frac{1}{H_{dC}} + \frac{X_W}{K_W} + \frac{1}{H_{dH}} + \frac{1}{H_H}$$

As the individual heat transfer coefficients increase, the overall heat transfer coefficient (U_o) increases. Fouling of either surface decreases the U_o. The fouling that occurs on the heat transfer fluid side of the vessel is usually caused by boiler steam scale or scale from untreated cooling water. This can be corrected by regular cleaning of the vessel jacket, and by use of water additives to minimize scaling.

The fouling that occurs on the process fluid side of the vessel is caused by buildup of the product due to its own viscosity and lack of turbulence (mixing) which makes this "boundary layer" thicker, preventing good heat transfer. The factors H_{dH} and H_{dC} are referred to as "film coefficients." There are thin layers of fluid that are in immediate contact with the surfaces of the vessel, both on the process side and the heat transfer fluid side. These thin layers represent the "film," which is essentially at rest. The film coefficient is a measure of the thermal conductivity through this resting fluid.

The importance of mixing as a unit operation is clearly demonstrated by its effect on the product film coefficient, H_{dC}. Higher mixing decreases the thickness of this film layer and permits more rapid heat transfer between the surface of the vessel and the bulk product. During heating, the film can be lower in viscosity than the product, which will improve heat transmission. It is during cooling that the product is subject to a significant decrease in heat transmission due to the increase in viscosity at the cool surface of the vessel. The mixing speed may need to be increased in order to produce the turbulence necessary to make the film thinner so that the bulk can be cooled at a satisfactory rate. The increased shear may be detrimental to the product, which may force a tradeoff between cooling rate and shear rate. A side-wiping agitator can remove this film and replace the cold bulk with warm fresh bulk to be cooled. The removal of the cold layer is of prime importance in providing the proper shear in mixing as well as the specified cooling rate. The relationship between mixing and heat transfer is important information needed for scale-up.

The mass transfer coefficient has a mathematical form similar to the heat transfer coefficient. Its units are in kilogram moles per square meter second in the MKS system. Qualitatively, it is a measure of how much mass is transferred per unit of available surface per second. The heat transfer coefficient is a measure of how much heat is transferred per unit of available surface per second. The driving force for heat transfer is the temperature gradient, ΔT. The driving force for mass transfer is ΔC, the concentration gradient. Mixing influences both in the same way. The formulation team must consider both when developing and scaling a process.

4. Types of Reactors and Their Use in Cosmetics

The most frequently used "reactor" in the cosmetics industry is the CSTR, or continuous stirred tank reactor. This is typically a jacketed stainless-steel vessel with agitation provided by propeller blade, anchor blade, side-wipe, homogenizer, or any combination of these. This type of reactor is used in batch processing. Jacketing the vessel allows a heat transfer medium (cooling water, glycol, steam, hot water, etc.) to circulate. Heat transfer is accomplished by conduction from the inner surface of the vessel, which is heated or cooled by the medium, to the batch. Mixing the batch in the vessel increases the efficiency of heat transfer by forced convection. In batch processing, all raw materials are added to the vessel in a specified order, and the reaction mixture should be homogeneous after each operation. Ideally, each incremental sample of the batch, from any location, should be the same as all others. Proper mixing will ensure homogeneity of the batch (mass transfer) as well as efficient heating or cooling.

In **semi-continuous or continuous processes**, it is more common to use a "plug flow reactor." Also called a pipeline reactor, it resembles just that. Unlike the CSTR, the contents of the pipe are not homogeneous throughout the length. Each incremental cross-section of the pipe is different in concentration (contents), and in temperature, from all others. Heat transfer in this type of process is attained by use of a jacket around the pipe similar to the CSTR. Increments of the pipe are heated or cooled as required by the process. As each increment, or plug, moves along the pipe it is subjected to a different set of concentration and temperature conditions. Each increment is homogeneous within itself, but is different from all others along the pipe.

Batch reactors are suitable for use in small-scale operations using expensive raw materials. This is more typical of the cosmetics industry where quality control is performed on a discrete batch-to-batch basis. When deviations occur, they occur in a particular batch and can be easily isolated. Continuous processes lend themselves to large-scale operations. When deviations occur, they can be harder to isolate and correct due to the overall variations along the reactor. Both systems require instrumentation to record and control process parameters. The batch-process parameters to measure and control are heat/cool rate and times, mixing speeds and times, and degree of vacuum (if a vacuum kettle is used).

Plug-flow reactor parameters to measure are rates of addition (to measure and control concentrations at any point in the pipe), temperature at each critical point in the reactor, mixing speeds (if dynamic pipeline mixing is used), pH, viscosity, conductivity (for complex emulsion systems), pressure/vacuum, and overall rate/product formation. The plug-flow reactor makes up for its advantages by requiring precise measurement and control devices, as well as alarms to alert operators to process variations. The choice of the particular reactor type depends on quantity of product to be made, complexity of formulation, sensitivity to reaction parameters of heat and mass transfer, fluid flow, and regulatory issues (e.g., over-the-counter, or OTC, drugs versus non-drug product).

5. Emulsion Processing Equipment—Heat Transfer

The most common heat transfer method used in the cosmetic industry is jacketing of a vessel/pipe. The jacket may be used for either heating or cooling with steam, water, or other heat transfer medium (specially designed oils and glycols). Most liquid products can be made using this type of cooling regardless of viscosity. Because of the necessity to mix the batch uniformly, excess mixing may occur during long cooling cycles, which can cause viscosity and stability variations.

It is important in scale-up to keep the overall heating and cooling rates the same through the changes in batch size. In heating, manufacturing will typically use steam. It is not recommended that the steam pressure on the kettle be higher than 15 psig (pounds per square inch gauge, or 1 bar). Saturated steam at a pressure of 15 psig creates a jacket and kettle wall temperature of 250°F (121°C). Steam pressures greater than 15 psig produce higher temperatures. The higher temperatures could cause degradation of ingredients on the walls of the kettle (particularly oxidation at the liquid-air interface). Other than the issue of burning material—cooling is typically a more critical process than heating. This is particularly true of emulsion products or products containing waxes. If this type of product is cooled in the laboratory in 20 minutes but requires a cooling time of 120 minutes in manufacturing, the resultant batches will not be identical. The microstructure of the emulsion or waxes could be totally different, affecting viscosity, feel, absorption, appearance and/or stability.

To overcome this problem, colder cooling media will be used in manufacturing than in the laboratory. The problem caused by this solution is that the product will be exposed to a much colder temperature at the wall of the kettle. This can result in premature solidification of waxes. To determine whether this is a concern or not, batches should be made in the laboratory or pilot plant using both fast and slow cooling rates.

Tube-and-shell or plate-and-frame heat exchangers can be used with some low-viscosity products, which are sensitive to shear. The larger ratio of surface area of cooling to product volume inherent in the design of this equipment allows heat transfer to be achieved quickly and efficiently. Only testing on the pilot or production scale will determine whether the product can acceptably be processed by this method. There are no simple laboratory systems available. Heating or cooling media, supply hopper, product transfer pump, and the heat exchanger must all be designed to work together for the product.

Products that are viscous can be pumped through a scraped-wall heat exchanger, Figure 13.5. This piece of equipment has a surface area to volume ratio that is less than the last two pieces discussed, but can provide cooling at rates four times or more than those in a continuous stirred tank reactor (CSTR). The disadvantage is that it can add considerable work to the product at lower temperatures. If the product requires a faster cool than can be achieved in a CSTR, and it can withstand shear at lower temperatures, the scraped-wall heat exchanger may be the process equipment of choice. Other heat exchanger designs are available; some are more compact or of sanitary design, which aids in the cleaning and sanitization process.

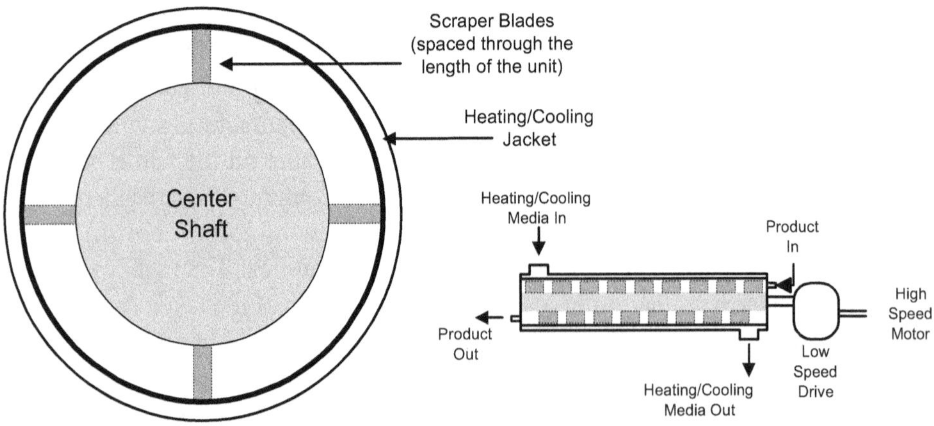

Figure 13.5: Scraped-wall heat exchanger

13.1.3.1 WET SYSTEMS—SINGLE PHASE (MISCIBLE) SYSTEMS

The science of mixing is far from complete. Designers of mixing equipment are not yet able to produce, from simple design principles, the optimum piece of equipment for a specific job even if they are given the necessary parameters and fundamental characteristics of the process and formula. One of the reasons for this is that the complete mathematical description of the flow pattern of fluid within each mixing vessel is extremely complex and difficult to achieve. Progress, however, is being made using the mathematical tools of dimensional analysis and modeling [4, 5, 6, and 7]. As an illustration of the practical usefulness of the data that can emerge from this analytical approach, a brief description of the relationship between some of the relevant parameters follows.

a. Flow Patterns: Fluids with Low or Medium Viscosity (< 5,000 centipoise)

Flow patterns in agitated vessels can be resolved into three principal types: tangential flow, radial flow, and axial flow.

In ***tangential flow***, the liquid moves parallel to the direction of the impeller. Movement of liquid into the surroundings is small and there is little movement perpendicular to the blades except in eddies near the tips. Tangential flow may be observed in paddle mixers operating at low speeds or in liquids of sufficient viscosity to prevent centrifugal flow from being developed, Figure 13.6a.

During ***radial flow***, the liquid is discharged outwards from the impeller by centrifugal force. If the moving liquid strikes the wall of the vessel, it splits into two sections, circulating back towards the impeller where it is re-entrained. The splitting of the flow at the wall induces further turbulence and mixing. There is usually some element of radial flow in all stirred vessels, but flat-blade turbines and disks with radial paddle blades or teeth are specifically designed to produce flow patterns that are primarily radial, Figure 13.6b.

Axial flow, as the name implies, takes place parallel to the axis of rotation. Usually the impeller or propeller blades are pitched so that liquid is discharged axially—the direction of flow may be from top to bottom of the vessel or vice versa, Figure 13.6c. Generally speaking the most difficult flow pattern to maintain is one of axial flow.

By far the most common form of mixing in liquids of low or medium viscosity (< 5,000 centipoise) is achieved by forced convection in stirred vessels. The motion of the liquid produced in the vessel must be sufficiently intense to sustain turbulence. Since it is unlikely that turbulence can be generated uniformly throughout the whole content of the vessel on the production scale, the liquid must be circulated continuously around the vessel so that all of it passes through those regions where turbulence develops. Thus, the number of important basic mixing parameters to be considered is two: the extent of turbulence, and the circulation rate of the contents.

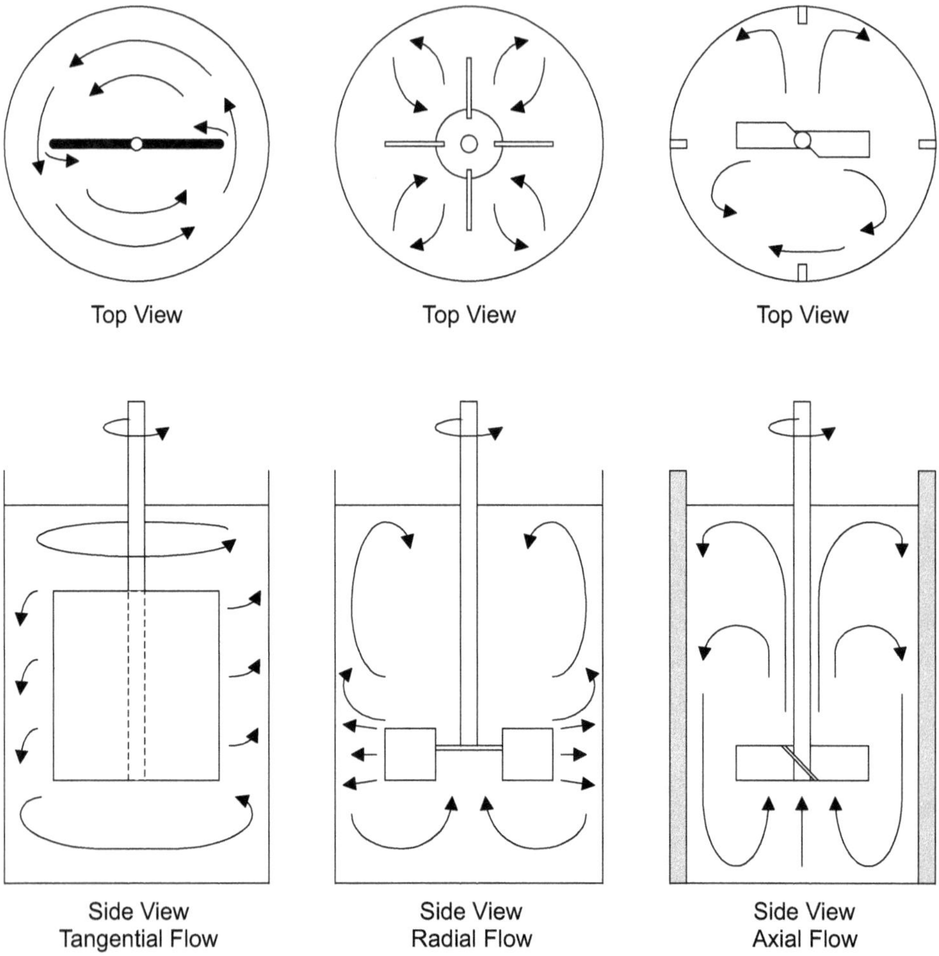

(a) (b) (c)

(a) tangential, around the circumference of the vessel

(b) radial, centrifugal off the peripheral tips of the blade

(c) axial, in the direction of the impeller shaft (baffles in vessel)

Figure 13.6: Flow patterns with different agitators

Viscous liquids showing shear-thinning characteristics present considerable problems to the cosmetics processor. The fluid close to the rotating impeller of a mixer is sheared at a high rate and so becomes relatively mobile. But as this is pumped away from the impeller, regions of less intense flow and hence of much higher viscosity are encountered. Turbulence is rapidly damped out, decreasing the turnover in the vessel and slowing down the mixing process. Scraper blades are often included on an anchor sweep, or contra-sweep to ensure good agitation along the vessel walls as the batch viscosity increases during cooling.

b. Impellers for Liquids of Low and Medium Viscosity

Paddle mixers produce mainly tangential flow and are usually mounted centrally because of their large diameter compared with that of the tank. For viscous liquids, the paddle is often of an anchor design equipped with scraper blades that remove product from the walls of the vessel.

Marine type ***Propeller mixers***, Figure 13.7a, are restricted to use with low-viscosity fluids, since their pumping capacity becomes localized at viscosities above 5000 centipoise. They have pitched blades whose angle varies along the length from center to tip. Flow patterns developed by propeller mixers have a high axial component and the rate of circulation around the vessel is high. Though the ideal impeller diameter to tank diameter ratio (D/T) is 0.33 ± 0.05, propeller mixers are usually of relatively small diameter, typically three-bladed, and are used at speeds between 150 to 2500 RPM. Such stirrers are used extensively in the cosmetics industry for simple blending operations. Alternate propeller mixer designs are available. These are commonly called **axial flow impellers**.

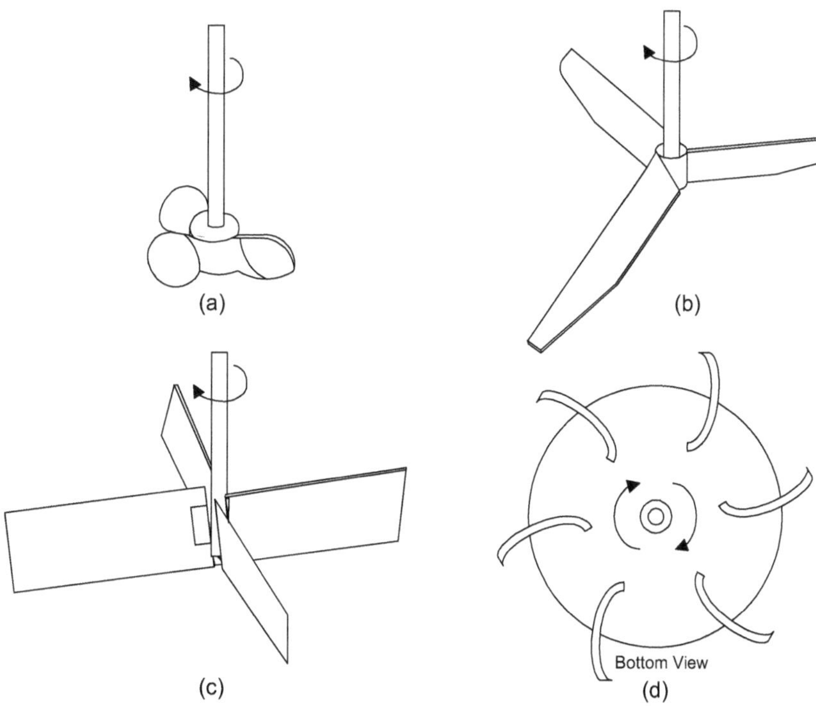

Figure 13.7: Designs of turbine impeller

Many portable mixers are of the propeller type. If the mixer is mounted centrally in the mixing tank, Figure 13.8 a, the surface becomes depressed and a vortex is formed. This is because of the natural movement of liquid to be drawn from above the impeller and towards its center. Generally, vortices are to be avoided because of the low order of turbulence and likely air-entrapment. Thus, propeller mixers should be mounted eccentrically, that is, offset from the center of the vessel at an angle other than perpendicular to the batch surface, Figure 13.8 b. Offset propeller mounting improves mixing efficiency by eliminating vortices, increasing turbulence, and improving batch turnover in the vessel. If the mixer must be mounted centrally, an alternate method of minimizing the formation of a vortex is through the addition of baffles, Figure 13.8 c. The baffles are normally equally spaced (e.g., four at 90° separations) and fixed to the vessel walls for efficiency. To improve ease of cleaning of the vessel, the baffles may not be fixed, but they then will not be sized the same to maintain the flow pattern required.

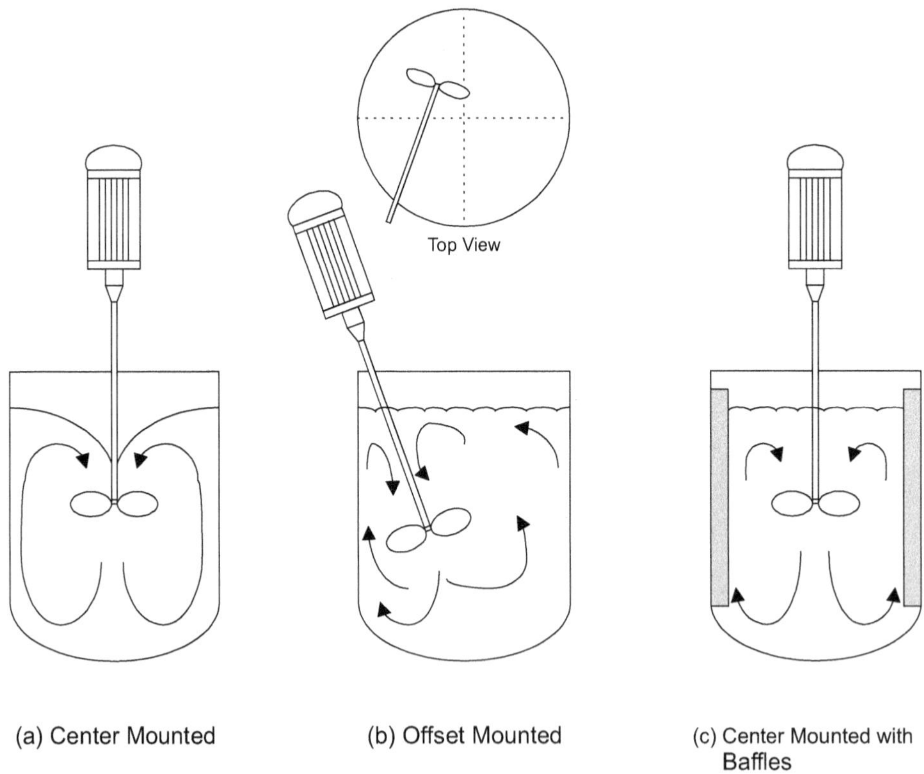

Figure 13.8: Portable mixer positioning

A *turbine prop* is a common impeller type used in cosmetics processing since it can cope with a wide range of viscosity and density. For liquids of low-viscosity, the flat-blade, axial-flow impeller is sometimes used, Figure 13.7 b. Slightly more viscous fluids are more efficiently mixed using the axial-flow flat-blade turbine shown in Figure 13.7 c. For very viscous materials, multiple radial-flow turbine blades, curved backwards in the direction opposite to the rotation, may be used, Figure 13.7 d. These require a lower starting torque and seem to give better energy transfer from impeller to liquid. Turbines produce a large flow of liquid with minimal shear and horsepower. They are normally mounted perpendicular to the top of the vessel with three or four baffles attached to the vertical vessel wall to reduce tangential and radial flow. Baffles help to induce and control the flow in both axial and radial directions. Used without baffles, the axial component generated by turbines remains secondary to the radial flow component, and the turbine does not efficiently turn over the entire batch. Typically, impellers of this kind are used at rotational speeds of 100 to 2000 revolutions per minute (RPM) as compared to the low speeds of 15 to 50 RPM for paddles.

c. Power Consumption

Power consumption is of great relevance to the economics of the mixing process. The choice of the wrong equipment can lead to the consumption of vastly greater quantities of power than are necessary to achieve the desired end result. On the other hand, sufficient power must be available and applied to the fluid to ensure that the endpoint of the mixing process can be achieved in a sensible time [5, 6, and 7].

As can be seen in Equation 13.6, a change in impeller diameter has a more significant effect on the power required than a change in impeller speed. This is emphasized in the design of most drop-in homogenizers through their small head design powered by a large drive motor.

$$P \propto \mathrm{N}^3\ \mathrm{D}^5$$

Where: P = Power in watts

N = Impeller Speed in revolutions per minute

D = Impeller Diameter in meters

Equation 13.6 Power relationship to impeller speed and diameter

d. Pumping Capacity and Velocity Head

Perhaps the most powerful concept to arise from the analytical approach to mixing concerns the way that power provided by each type of impeller is actually transmitted to the fluid. This relationship can be expressed generally as

$$P \propto Q\,H$$

Where: P = Power in watts

Q = Pumping Capacity in liters per minute

H = Velocity Head in meters

Equation 13.7 Power relationship to pumping capacity and velocity head

Q is the pumping capacity of the impeller (the volume of fluid displaced directly by the impeller in liters per minute) and H is the velocity head—this is related to the shear rate experienced by fluid leaving the impeller. A large slow-moving impeller might produce, for example, a large pumping capacity and a low-velocity head, while a small impeller operating at high speed might produce a lower volume of fluid pumping but at a much higher-velocity head. Most cosmetics production processes require high pumping capacity, while others require high shear rate. It is useful to know the parameters that affect both these functions and how they interrelate.

For simple blending operations (the manufacture of shampoos or colognes, for example) pumping capacity of the impeller is often of the greatest significance. Under conditions of laminar flow, the number of complete changes of the bulk (batch turnover) required to bring about homogeneity is approximately three. For a turbine operating in turbulent conditions, this is reduced to about 1.5. However, given that only a fixed amount of power is available from the motor, it is not likely that a relatively small turbine will have sufficient pumping capacity to push a fairly viscous product around by even this amount. Not surprisingly, the factor that determines whether power is used as pumping capacity or velocity head is the ratio of impeller to tank diameter (D/T).

Examining the relationship between power consumption and D/T ratio for equal process results in a given vessel completes the picture, Figure 13.9. The use of a D/T ratio larger than 0.6 lowers the power required to achieve the same end result. At the same time, this implies the use of lower impeller speed, and this inevitably means that the torque required to drive the mixer increases dramatically [8]. The amount of torque that a given mixer is able to generate depends largely on its construction. It becomes a question of economics whether to invest in a more substantial (and expensive) mixer in order to reduce the power consumption needed to achieve a given mixture quality.

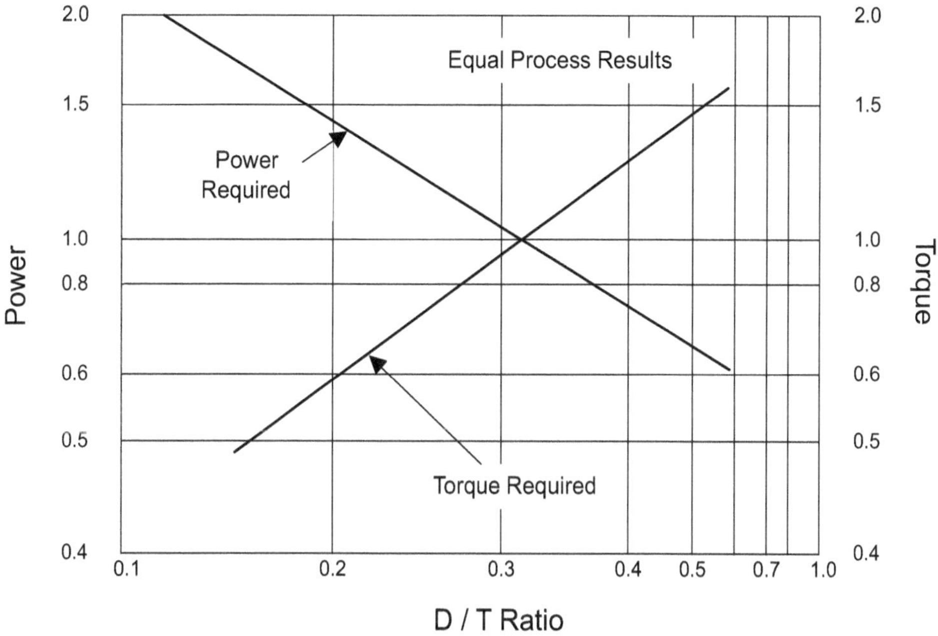

Figure 13.9 Power and torque relationship for equal process results [9]

e. Mixing Time

Another important measurable parameter is mixing time, t_m. This is the time taken to achieve the desired degree of homogeneity in the mixture. There are many methods by which this characteristic may be measured, but perhaps the most obvious is the time taken for a soluble dye to become uniformly dispersed throughout the mixing vessel (e.g., in the manufacture of a colored shampoo). The relationship between mixing time, t_m, and the degree of uniformity can clearly be shown if some index of mixing level can be established.

A simple example of this would be the ratio of color intensity between the top and bottom of the vessel contents at intervals after dye is added to the top (so that uniformity is achieved as the mixing index, M, approaches unity). This comparatively simple experiment should give rise to a curve similar to that shown in Figure 13.10. Since the approach of M to unity is asymptotic, t_m is difficult to measure accurately unless a colorimeter or other optical measuring device is available.

Once t_m has been established, however, more useful insight into the parameters controlling mixing rates may be gleaned from relationships such as that illustrated in Figure 13.11 [5, 6, 7, and 10]. In Figure 13.11a (which relates to a viscous liquid in which turbulence is not established), t_m, the mixing time, has been replaced by the product of rotational speed N and t_m, that is, by the number of revolutions of the impeller. M, the mixing index, has been replaced by log (1-M) to present the plot in a linear fashion.

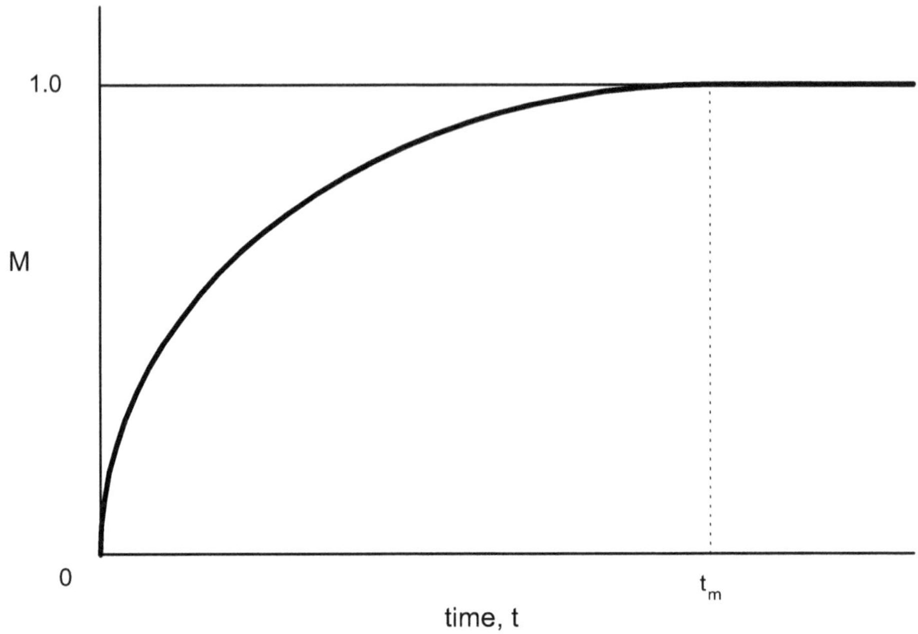

Figure 13.10 Mixing index, M, plotted against time to give mixing time, t_m

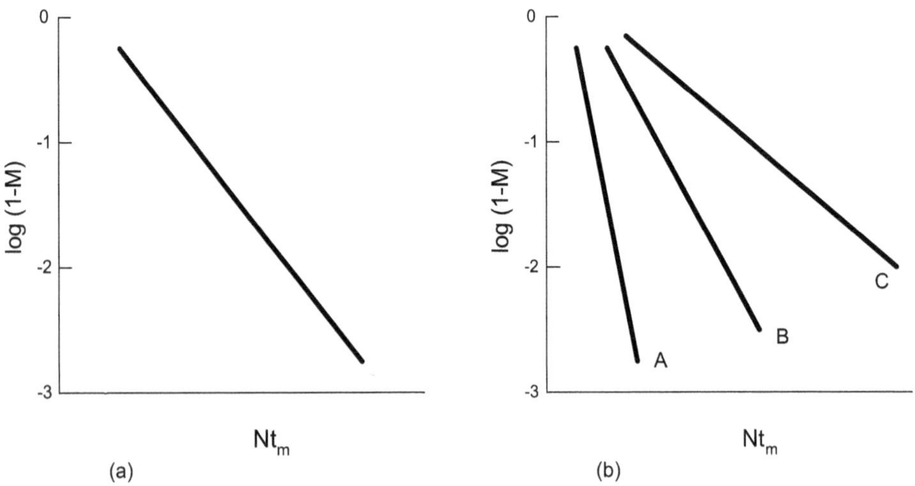

Figure 13.11: Mixing index, M, plotted against number of revolutions, Nt_m
(a) Newtonian fluids (b) non-Newtonian fluids

It is interesting to note that for Newtonian fluids (ideal response between stress and strain) precisely the same plot is produced whatever the viscosity of the medium and speed of the impeller. In other words, only the number of impeller revolutions determines the change in mixing index. This is not true of non-Newtonian fluids—plots A, B, and C in Figure 13.11 b, which represents liquids showing increasing divergence from Newtonian behavior. This illustrates the difficulties of mixing non-Newtonian media in which flow is damped out rapidly by regions of high viscosity away from the vicinity of the impeller blade.

f. Influence of Vessel Shape

The ratio of tank dimensions can be an important factor in determining the efficiency of any mixing process. It is sensible to perform a simple blending, such as alcohol-water, in tall cylindrical vessels of small cross-section using a propeller or turbine mixer with two or three sets of blades located two to three blade diameters apart on the same shaft. This stirred tank setup allows the capability to make variable batch volumes with high axial flow. For low-viscosity lotions, a hemispherical kettle often replaces the dished bottom conical tank to maximize the batch turnover achieved with an offset-mounted propeller mixer. Normally the ratio of kettle diameter to kettle height is close to 1:1. In the production of an emulsion of medium viscosity, it is desirable to keep the height of the vessel between 1 and 1.5 times its diameter.

g. Flow Patterns: Fluids of High Viscosity

As the viscosity of the mixture increases, it becomes increasingly difficult—and eventually mechanically impossible—to produce turbulent flow within the mixing vessel. At viscosities of 100,000 centipoise or above, flow is inevitably laminar, power consumption high, and the rate of mixing exceedingly low. In such systems, the input power should be used to create disorder (mixing) but is used to create heat. The rate of temperature rise is dependent upon the energy input, the thermal conductivity of the mixture, and the efficiency of the cooling surfaces; but the range 1° to 3°C per minute would include many cosmetic mixing processes of this kind.

Generally it is difficult or impossible during industrial mixing of highly viscous materials to dissipate heat faster than it is generated. This is particularly true if the mixing vessel is of large capacity (in which the ratio of volume to heat-exchange surface is high) and if appreciable films of chilled liquid are allowed to build up on the walls of the vessel, so insulating the contents from further cooling. The increase in temperature associated with such processes has both advantages and disadvantages. On the one hand a rise in temperature might cause a decrease in viscosity, making mixing more efficient, and might also help in the melting or dissolution of some of the components of the mixture. Taken too far, on the other hand, the decrease in shear stress caused by the fall in viscosity can decrease the efficiency of stress-dependent processes. This can be seen when breaking up and dispersing pigment agglomerates. The increase in temperature may damage the product by causing the thermal degradation of heat-sensitive components such as actives, preservatives, and perfumes. The relatively high-energy input required while mixing viscous materials also influences the mechanical construction of the mixing machinery and the method by which mixing is achieved.

h. Impeller Types and Mixers for High-Viscosity Fluids

Propellers and turbines, as already mentioned, work best under turbulent conditions at relatively high rotational speeds. In viscous products (given that such speeds are attainable at all), flow is confined to the regions very close to the impeller. Large stagnant regions in the vessel exist where no mixing can occur without the employment of some secondary mechanism. To eliminate these stagnant regions large impellers such as paddles, gates, anchors, and leaf impellers may be used. These sweep a much greater proportion of the vessel and produce more extensive flow. Usually such impellers are designed to have close clearances with walls, giving a degree of wall scraping. This helps to eliminate buildup of unmixed materials at the walls, provides a region of high shear for dispersing aggregates and lumps, and may improve the wall heat transfer to and from the bulk.

Such impellers provide extensive flow but only of the tangential and radial variety. Axial flow, and therefore top-to-bottom mixing, is almost totally absent. This is a limitation of the design. Several suppliers have developed agitation techniques that include special baffles (often of variable pitch) that induce flow in both the downward and upward directions. For this reason, recycling the batch either externally through a pump or with time using the pitch of the sweep blade becomes an important consideration.

An alternative approach to the problem created by lack of flow in viscous media is the use of impellers that progressively sweep the whole contents of the vessel while the mixture remains stationary. Examples of this include the mixer in which a helical screw sweeps the wall of a conical mixing chamber, Figure 13.12. Equipment that exhibits a greater degree of distributive mixing may be utilized for more viscous products such as mascaras and toothpastes. Such mixers are designed to produce bulk flow and laminar shear by spatial redistribution of elements of the mixture. Perhaps the most commonly encountered mixers of this type are of the single or double action planetary type or the two-blade "dough" mixer. Their essential feature involves the cutting and folding of a volume of the mixture and the physical replacement of it into another part of the mixture where it is cut and folded again.

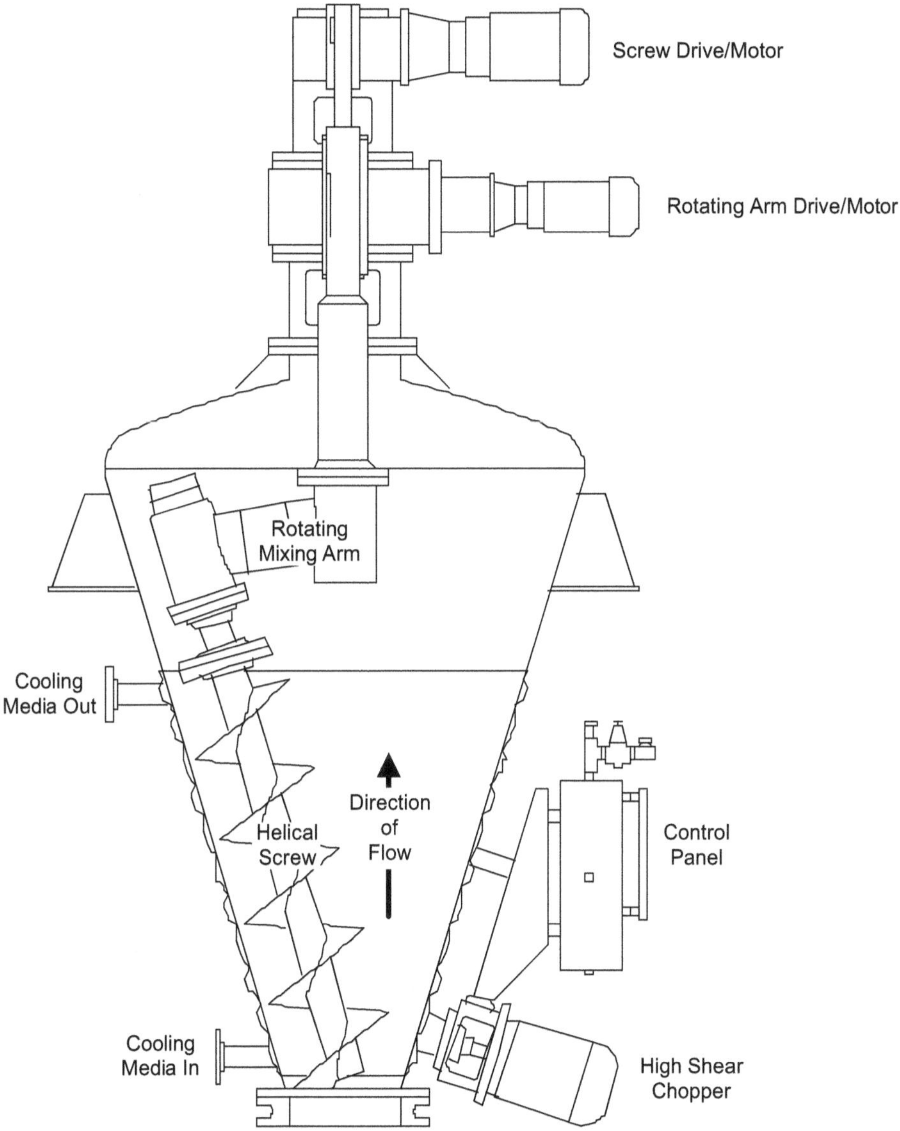

Figure 13.12: High solids blender [11]
Figure Courtesy of Charles Ross and Son Company, Hauppauge, New York

The static mixer is essentially an in-line mixing device in which mixtures flowing through a pipe are cut and folded by a series of helical elements in a circular tube, Figure 13.13. These elements (which do not move—hence the name "static") turn the flowing mixture through an angle of 180°. Since alternate elements have opposite pitch and are displaced 90° to each other, this causes the bulk flow to reverse direction at each junction. The leading edge of each element becomes a cutting device, splitting and refolding the mixture in and on itself. This type of static mixer works well with thick materials. Other static, or motionless, mixer designs utilize the divergence and convergence of flows to induce mixing with some control as to the shear developed. This type of static mixer works well with thin materials. It can be seen that with both high and low viscosities, excellent mixing can be achieved in a relatively short length of pipe and with relatively few static elements. Each element splits the product stream in two and combines the two new streams with parts of the previously split streams. Other styles of static mixers are also available that offer specialty features such as adjustable gap settings and lower pressure drops.

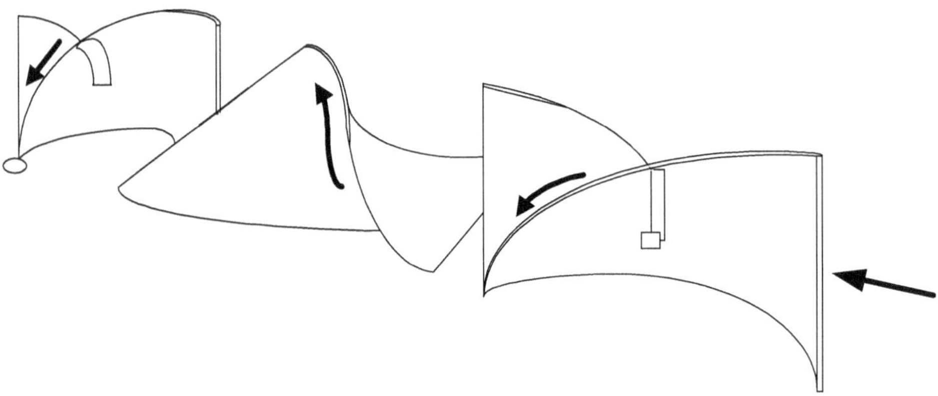

Figure 13.13: Static mixer elements

Finally, mention must be made of extruders, in which a helical screw forces the bulk mixture to flow down a tube. Here, the pressure generated can be enormous, as in soap plodding, and such energy can cause materials with high viscosity to undergo laminar flow and change structure. The actual flow pattern produced is complex, being a combination of pressure and drag flow within the tube [12].

13.1.3.2 WET SYSTEMS - MULTIPHASE SYSTEMS

a. The Emulsification Process

Two major immiscible phases (referred to as "oil" and "water") together with the emulsifier are brought together to form an emulsion. If the chemistry is favorable, very little energy is needed to produce a stable product. To minimize the level of emulsifier, it may be possible to use energy to force the emulsion to a stable end-point.

The level of energy required will be formula dependent. Under turbulent conditions, one phase (usually the discontinuous or internal phase) is broken up into droplets (predominantly by the action of shear stress imparted by turbulent eddies). The droplets are distributed throughout the other phase (the continuous or external phase).

While the droplets remain larger than the majority of the flowing particles, they will continue to break up into ever-smaller droplets. Eventually a point is reached in this process when the available power creating the turbulence cannot provide the shear stress necessary to reduce the droplet size any further. At this stage an emulsion exists containing droplets of a certain mean diameter ranging from d_{min} to d_{max}. Provided that it is correctly chosen, the emulsifier prevents the rapid coalescence of these droplets, and a stable emulsion may be formed.

In order to obtain products of maximum stability that can be made consistently from batch to batch, it is generally desirable to keep the droplet size distribution as narrow as possible. In a CSTR, droplet size is smallest near the impeller in the region of greatest turbulence whereas the maximum droplet size is to be found in any quiescent region of the tank. Thus it can be seen that d_{min} is fixed by the power available to generate turbulence, and d_{max} depends on the efficiency of the mixing in the tank to produce a good circulation rate, to bring all the contents through the region of maximum turbulence. This will minimize the distribution range between d_{min} and d_{max}.

Superimposed on the effect of circulation patterns in the vessel is an additional factor affecting the particle size range of the droplets. For a given vessel and impeller the effect of increasing the mixer speed should be to reduce the particle size range to a minimum, after which a further increase in speed could give rise to instability and coalescence. In practice, coalescence does not take place if a sufficient quantity of emulsifier is present; nevertheless it is important to attain the correct impeller speed to reduce the particle size range to a minimum.

b. Orientation of Phases

In any emulsion the orientation of the phases (that is, whether the oil or the water phase is continuous) is determined principally by the choice of emulsifier and the volume ratio of oil to water. Usually there is a range of volume ratios over which either phase may be dispersed, depending upon the method of manufacture.

Initially, only one phase is present in the mixing vessel containing the impeller. The second phase will form the dispersed or discontinuous phase upon its addition. If the second phase is combined with the choice of emulsifier, which eventually leads to a volume ratio at which the system is more stable with the second phase being continuous, then the emulsion will spontaneously invert and the continuous and discontinuous phases will switch. When an inversion takes place, it is very often accompanied by an abrupt change in droplet size. Where this droplet size change is a decrease, the inversion leads to a more stable emulsion and gives rise to a valuable method of manufacture. This inversion process is often an effective method of producing a uniform, fine droplet size and may improve stability of the emulsion. Chemical formula, processing temperature, and energy must all combine at the correct levels for an inversion process to be reproducible in both the Laboratory and Production. Available energy level in Production is usually the limiting factor.

c. Addition of Surfactant

In a batch manufacturing process for emulsions, there are four possible methods of adding the emulsifier:

- dissolving or dispersing an emulsifying agent in water
- dissolving or dispersing an emulsifying agent in oil
- dissolving or dispersing an emulsifying agent in both the water and oil
- adding the water and oil phases alternately to an emulsifying agent

Normally, the emulsion process starts with a water phase to which the oil is added. An oil-in-water emulsion is initially produced, but an inversion to a water-in-oil emulsion may take place if sufficient oil is added. If the emulsifier is added to the oil phase, this mixture may be added directly to water to form an oil-in-water emulsion; if the water is added to the surfactant/oil mixture, a water-in-oil emulsion is formed initially.

Some emulsions are stabilized by "soaps," which are formed at the interface between the two phases. In this case, the fatty acid is dissolved in the oil and the alkaline component is dissolved in the water. The two phases can be brought together in any order. The neutralization reaction, which forms the emulsifier, takes place as the phases are combined.

A less-used method is one in which both the water and oil phases are added alternately to the emulsifying agent. Usually, the small improvement in product quality obtained by the use of this method does not warrant the complication it causes in the manufacturing procedure.

d. Emulsion Temperature

The primary reason for operating above room temperature during the manufacture of an emulsion is to ensure that both phases are in the liquid state. In particular, the oil phase may contain fats and waxes that are solid at room temperature. The water phase is customarily heated slightly above the temperature chosen for the oil phase so as not to cause any sudden solidification upon blending. There is, however, an interesting variation: emulsification between a hot oil phase and a cold (usually room temperature) water phase. An illustration of this procedure in which mixing and homogenization of the phases take place simultaneously is shown in Figure 13.14. The advantage of such a method is the saving of time and energy by not having to heat the aqueous phase and by reducing the time and energy required to cool the product to room temperature.

A secondary reason for heating a phase is to minimize microbiological concerns associated with a raw material. Preservatives are normally added to a formula to control any issues produced by the consumer. Minimizing growth can be performed in the process by using high-energy homogenizers (an inefficient use of the equipment) or by phase temperature (holding the phase at an elevated temperature for an extended period of time). A challenge when looking to move from a hot water/hot oil process to a cold water/hot oil process is whether or not the microbiology team supports the process change. It does not help to make batches quickly if they fail microbiological testing.

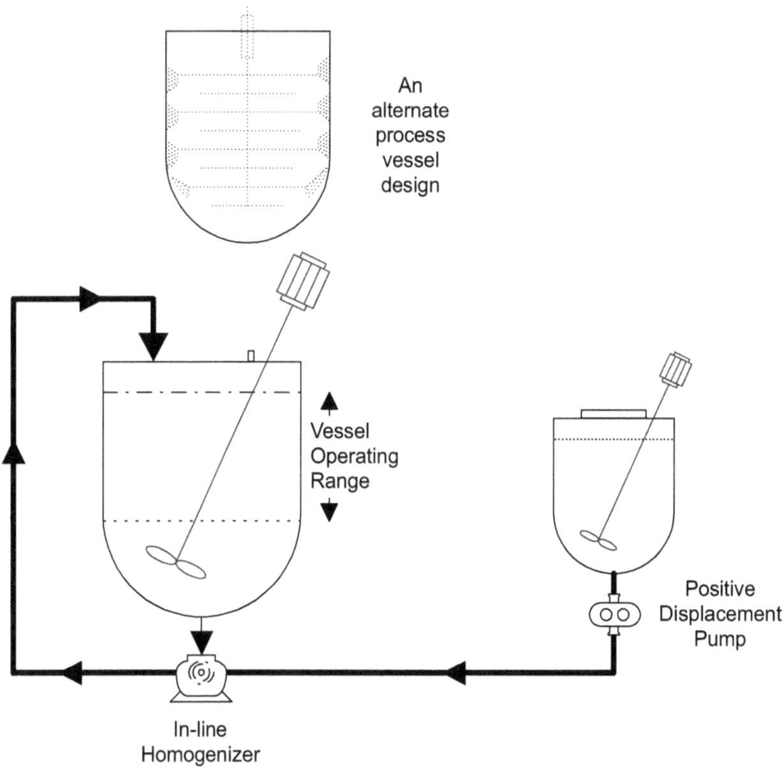

Figure 13.14: Hot/cold processing emulsion system

e. Emulsion Processing Equipment - Mixing

It is evident from the discussion so far that there are two important elements of emulsion processing: shear for emulsification and particle size reduction and flow for circulation of vessel contents through the region of maximum shear. Flow is also important in the heating and cooling of the emulsion. Most emulsion processing vessels are equipped with a jacket through which steam or hot water or cold/chilled water can be circulated for temperature control. To be effective, the mixing mechanism must include adequate flow to and from the vessel walls, as discussed earlier in this chapter.

For these reasons, most emulsion batch processing vessels contain a high-shear turbine or rotor-stator homogenizer (bottom, side, or top entry). High flow in one design, Figure 13.15, is provided by a paddle-style anchor agitator with scraper feet, which meshes with two fixed baffles (mating blades). The agitator can be run intermittently in either direction to provide a complete mix. In another design, Figure 13.16, concentric central shafts carry blades that turn in opposite directions and sweep the area in-between (counter-sweep). A frame holding the outer blades carries spring-loaded or product-pressure scraper blades to prevent buildup of product on the vessel wall, while mixing in the higher-viscosity region is thus enhanced. Mixing can be further enhanced by recirculation of the batch through the homogenizer and depositing it on the top of the batch to enhance plug flow. The recirculation piping may be an integral part of the vessel design (as shown in Figure 13.15) or an added feature in the production facility utilizing an external pump and piping (permanent line or hoses).

The need to combine all of these mixing capabilities into one vessel has led to the design shown in Figure 13.15. The following capabilities are available with no additional piping or equipment needed:

- Universal in application. It is capable of handling the entire viscosity range from light lotions to heavy ointments.
- Efficient presentation of the batch to the homogenizer for all batches. Efficient mixing ensures that all parts of the batch will see the same quantity of energy.
- Vacuum capable for maximum production efficiencies (high mixing speeds without aeration) and specific gravity control capabilities. Product integrity is not compromised during processing since aeration during mixing is not a factor.
- Clean-in-place and sanitize-in-place capable. The system is designed to be sanitary and maintain appropriate controls to meet the requirements for food, drug, and cosmetics manufacture.

Alternate designs are available from many suppliers in an effort to meet the above requirements (e.g., Figure 13.17). It is important for personnel purchasing equipment to understand the flexibility that is available in light of the processing requirements of new and upcoming products.

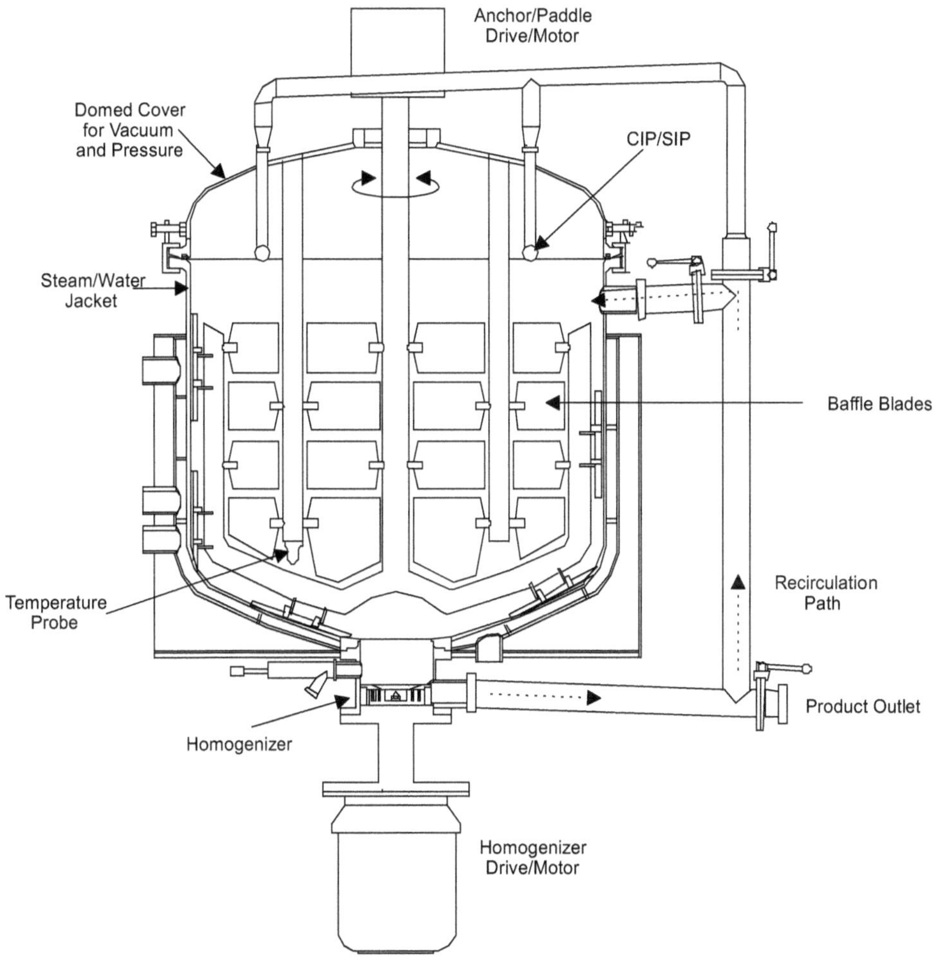

Figure 13.15: Batch emulsion processing vessel—SYMEX® Style - homogenizer in the down position [13];
Figure Courtesy of Schröder and Boos, Misch- & Anlagentechnik GmbH & Co. KG, Bremerhaven, Germany.

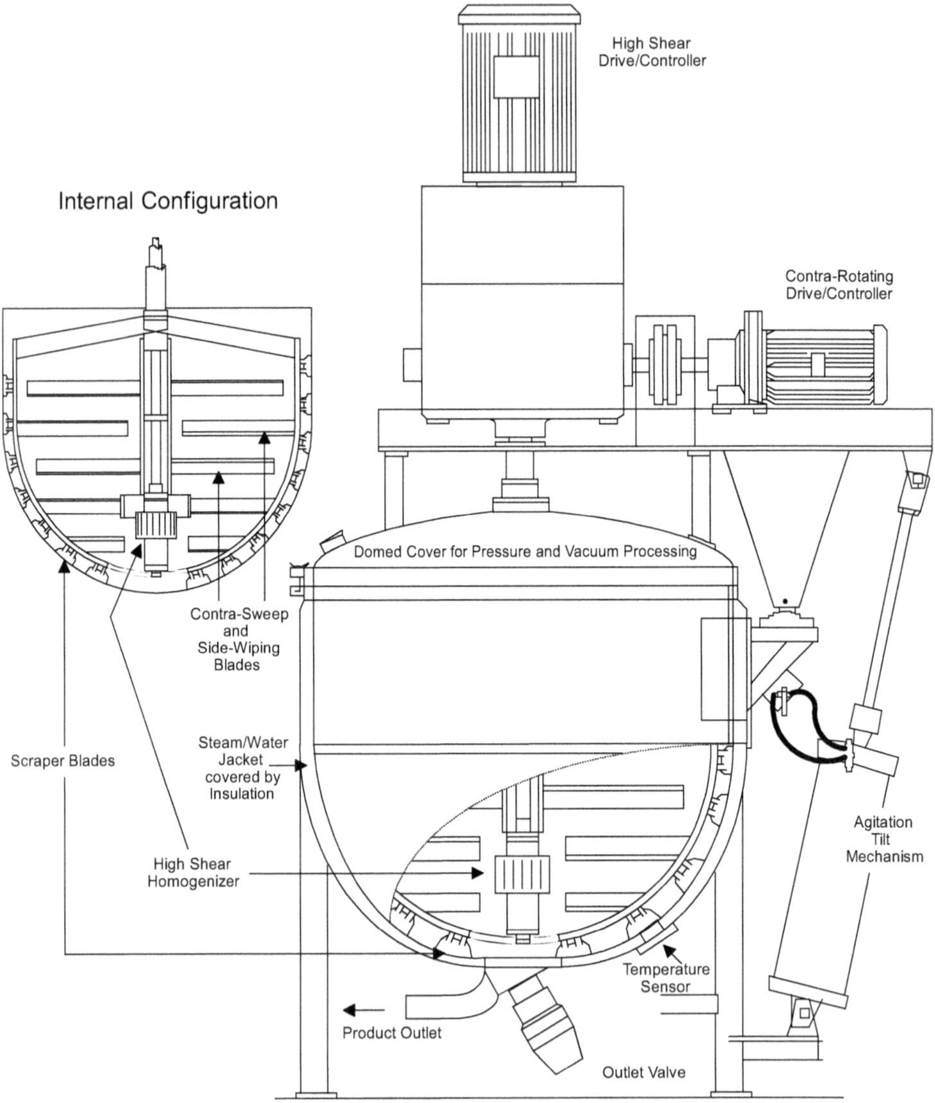

Figure 13.16: Batch Emulsion processing vessel—Lee® Tri-Mix Turbo-Shear® Style [14]
Figure Courtesy of Lee® Industries, Philipsburg, Pennsylvania.

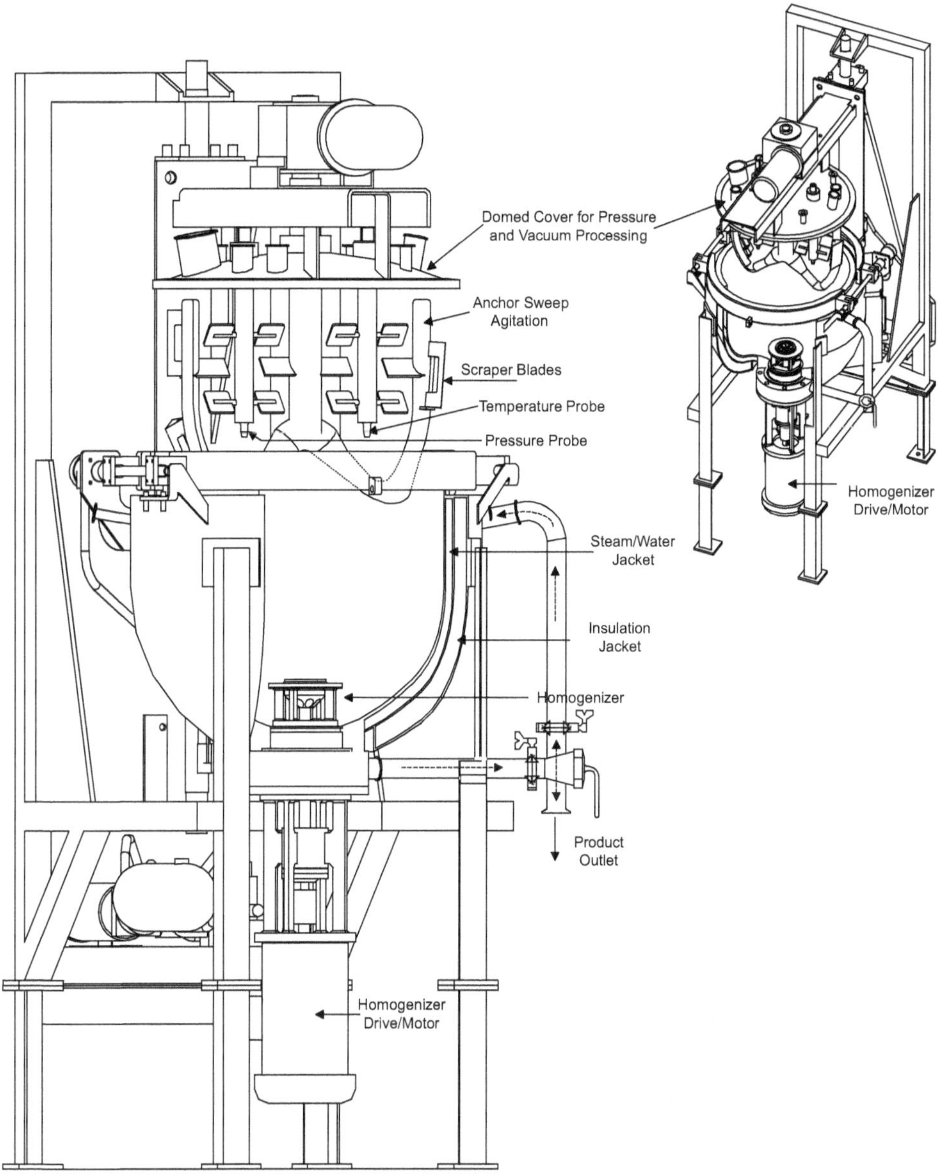

Figure 13.17: Batch emulsion processing vessel—AGI™ Mixer Triple Shaft, homogenizer in the up position [15]
Figure Courtesy of Chemineer®-Greerco®, North Andover, Massachusetts.

f. High-Shear Mixers and Dispersion Equipment

The mixing equipment that has so far been covered in this chapter is designed primarily to produce bulk flow patterns of sufficient intensity to allow mixing. In the majority of cases, the pattern of shear and turbulence developed within the mixture varies according to the viscosity of the bulk, the method of producing flow, and the volume within the mixture under consideration. For certain applications, however, it is desirable to generate a very intense degree of shear stress in the mixture, and for this purpose specialized equipment is available. The uses to which such machines are put in cosmetics processing include the breaking up of pigment agglomerates and their dispersion in liquids, the rapid fracture and dispersion of gelling agents (e.g., bentone clays, polymeric cellulose derivatives, and alginate-type polymers), and the size reduction of internal phase droplets in emulsion products.

g. Batch Homogenizers

All three types of batch homogenizers (top mounted, bottom mounted in the kettle with or without recirculation and in-line) operate under the same principles. Liquid is drawn into the inlet by the suction created by the rotating blades, or teeth, of the rotor (centrifugal force). The liquid is then forced through the stator configuration, subjecting the fluid to high mechanical shear at the rotor/stator interface. After the fluid exits the stator it is subjected to high hydraulic shear as it returns to the vessel or pipeline. The design of the rotor and the stator dictates the magnitude of shear stress developed by the homogenizer. *High-flow/low-shear homogenizers* normally employ a flat or pitched design with an open stator design, Figure 13.18 a. The stator will have slotted, round, or other discharge port configurations and discharges radially or axially.

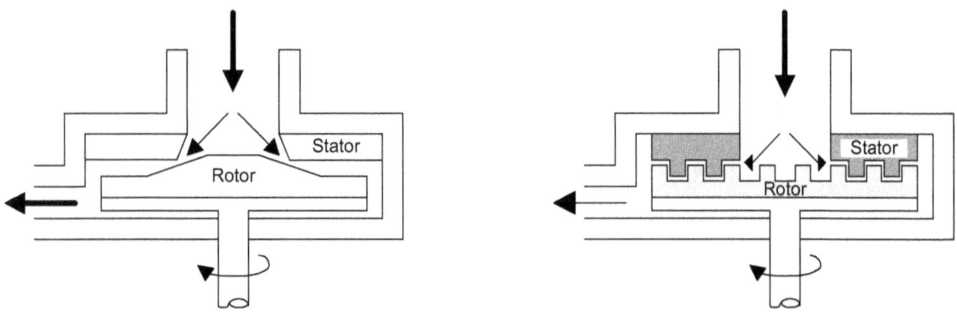

(a) High Flow Rotor/Stator Homogenizer

(b) Low Flow Rotor/Stator Homogenizer (Higher Shear)

Figure 13.18: Rotor/Stator designs

Major applications of the high-flow design are for traditional creams and lotions and other low- to medium-viscosity products where frequent particle interaction with low shear rates is required. High-shear/low-flow homogenizers are characterized typically by an intermeshing toothed rotor/stator design, Figure 13.18 b. The rotor and stator frequently have multiple rows of teeth, which operate at a gap range of 0.005"–0.015" (0.127–0.381 mm). The close tolerance increases the shear stress but has the effect of reducing the batch turnover rate. Major applications for this design are makeup pigment dispersion, mascara production, and low-emulsifier cream and lotion formulations that depend on mechanical energy for emulsification. Some vessels may allow interchangeability between high-flow/low-shear and high-shear/low-flow homogenizing heads. These units provide maximum flexibility for the production of a wide range of finished products ranging from thin lotions to thick ointments.

Some new designs provide additional flow and shear control through interchangeable slot configurations (a technique also used in laboratory homogenizers) and a rotor/stator design where both components can move in both directions. In theory, a wide range of flow rates and shear rates can be produced in one vessel using this new rotor/stator design.

A disadvantage of the top-entering homogenizer is the tendency of the mixer to cause aeration due to vortex formation—particularly when the homogenizer head is not completely covered. For this reason, high-shear devices are often incorporated into the bottom of the processing vessels. Additional advantages to the bottom-mounted design include the following: low-volume processing with minimal aeration, consistent agitation throughout the mass, virtually no minimum batch size, and fewer seal problems and less wear due to shorter shaft length. If the homogenizer is the primary mixer in the vessel, the outer tips of the rotor may wear rapidly, leading to increased clearance and decreased efficiency. Since no adjustment is possible, worn rotors must be replaced at considerable cost. Some designs also allow the homogenizer to be used as the discharge pump simplifying the total operation.

Generally, high-shear rotor-stator mixers may be used either for batch processing in a mixing tank (as a drop-in unit) or as in-line devices when encased in a suitable chamber. Used as batch mixers, they are capable of generating considerable turbulence because of the great velocity with which fluid is pumped out of the mixing head. In the high-viscosity region, pumping capacity decreases significantly. In this situation, use of an in-line device can be more effective. A positive displacement pump should be used to minimize viscosity effects during homogenization. The in-line homogenizer routinely has a significantly lower batch turnover rate than a drop-in homogenizer due to the restrictions of the recirculation arm, especially as batch sizes increase. This limitation may be overcome since it is highly effective as a finishing step for products during discharge. It should be remembered that mixing time is required to ensure that every part of the mixture has passed through the shear head at least once.

h. Continuous High-Pressure Homogenizers and Mixers

High-pressure homogenizers require a continuous process. This may be part of a recirculation line for a one-kettle operation or it may involve multiple kettles with a single pass or multiple passes through the device. The problems with most high-pressure systems are the high initial and operating costs and the low production-processing rate. The advantages lie in the small particle sizes that can be created during processing of both emulsions and solids dispersed in liquids.

Perhaps the highest shear stress is generated by the valve homogenizer, which is still extensively used in the production of emulsions with very fine internal phase droplets. A valve homogenizer, Figure 13.19, consists of a high-pressure pump, which forces product through a small orifice at pressures of up to 30,000 psi (2000 bar). Rapid expansion of the product after traveling through the orifice produces very fine emulsion and dispersion particles that are smaller than those produced by most other equipment.

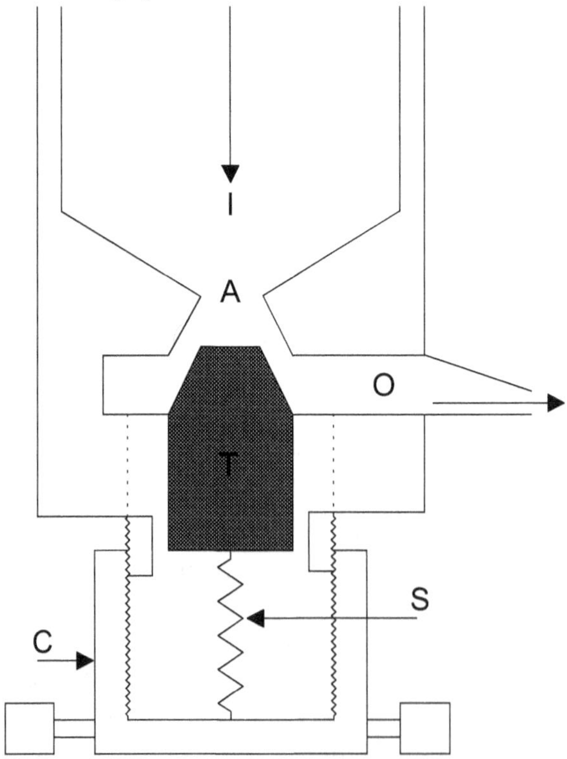

The roughly premixed product at I is forced through the valve seating at A and leaves via O. T is a tapered shaft whose position can be adjusted with screw head C. S is a powerful spring against which the product is pushed through the narrow valve orifice.

Figure 13.19: Valve homogenizer

An alternative to the valve homogenizer is the ultrasonic homogenizer. When high-intensity ultrasonic energy is applied to liquids, a phenomenon known as "cavitation" occurs. Cavitation is complex and not easily understood. As ultrasonic waves are propagated through the fluid, areas of compression and rarefaction are formed, and cavitation is produced in these rarefied areas. When the ultrasonic wave passes on, these cavities collapse and change to an area of compression. It has been demonstrated that the pressure in these cavities, just before their collapse, can be as high as several thousand bars. Most of the effects of ultrasonic homogenization in liquids are attributed to the powerful shock waves produced immediately following the collapse of such cavities. Units are available for both batch (like a drop-in homogenizer) and continuous processing. Most production systems will use the continuous or flow-through cell technology. One design of an ultrasonic homogenizer is illustrated in Figure 13.20. The energy developed through the cavitation process will wear specific components. These will need regular replacement to maintain process efficiency.

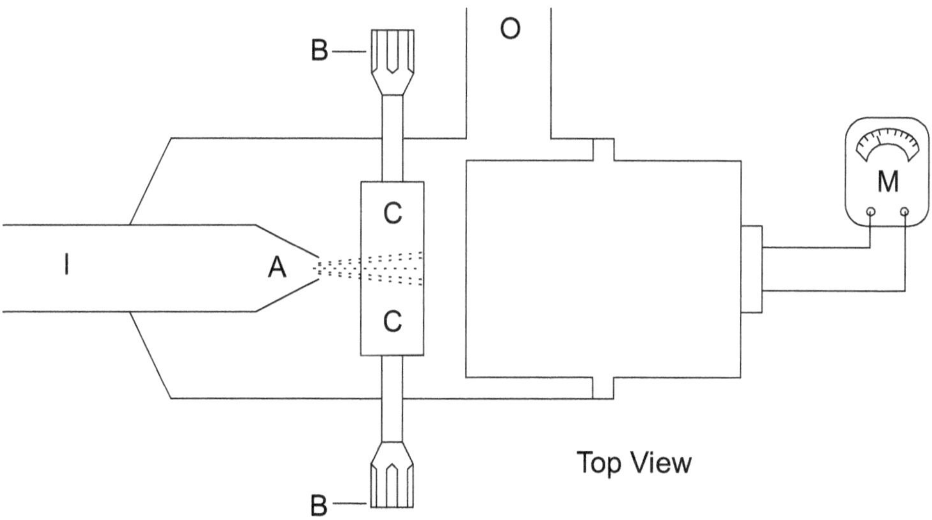

The roughly premixed product enters at I. It passes through orifice A and is subjected to intense ultrasonic energy by vibrating blade C. The treated product leaves via O. The meter, M, and "tuning" devices at B combine to allow the operator to maximize the settings for each product

Figure 13.20: Ultrasonic Homogenizer

A third alternative to the valve homogenizer is a design that forces fluid, at high pressure, through an orifice into an expansion and impingement chamber, Figure 13.21. These systems can usually achieve higher pressures than the other designs described, from 15,000 psi (1000 bar) up to 40,000 psi (2757 bar) and higher. These systems are often used in the processing of liposomes and special dispersions. Costs of these dispersions are high, and production flow rates are low.

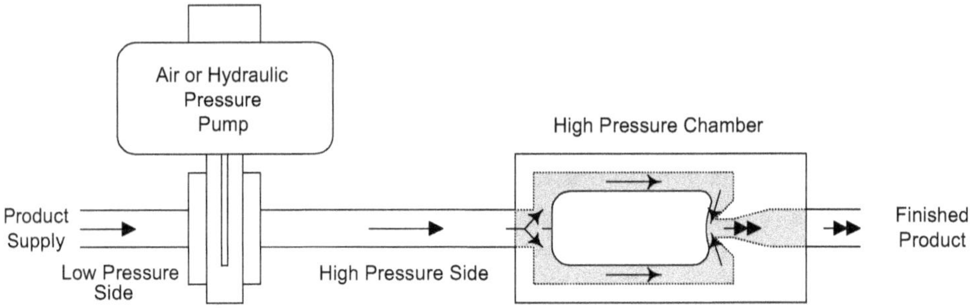

Figure 13.21: Multi-stream high-pressure homogenizer

i. Processing of Water in Silicone Emulsions

Advances in silicone technology have offered an alternative set of synthetic chemicals to the hydrocarbon compounds that have traditionally been used in the cosmetics industry, both as emulsifiers and as oil phase ingredients. In the case of emulsifiers, many specialty products can be derived by selective block copolymerization with hydrophilic materials along the siloxane backbone of the chain. The result of this block copolymerization is a molecule with a strongly hydrophobic Si-O-Si backbone with a 130° bond angle that allows a series of hydrophilic sites to rotate freely about that backbone with minimal steric restriction.

In working with silicone emulsifiers, described in great detail elsewhere in this book, the key processing step in forming a stable emulsion is allowing enough time for the randomly oriented hydrophilic sites to uncoil and become oriented to the water phase with the less polar and highly flexible Si-O-Si backbone following the curvature of a single water droplet. Failure to allow time for this orientation and coating action to progress to completion usually leads to a less stable emulsion that loses viscosity over time and can lead to syneresis (separation of the phases) as the water droplets coalesce. Thus, normal processing of water-in-silicone (W/S) emulsions involves introducing the water phase into the silicone phase very slowly with low-shear agitation to produce a "crude" emulsion that, after a mixing period, is "finished" by a high-shear mixing step. Failure to follow the above process can yield an emulsion that meets initial viscosity specifications and looks fine but deteriorates in two to four weeks into a low-viscosity product that may even bleed (syneresis).

Low-shear turbulent mixing can be accomplished with a turbine, sweep, or propeller blade turning with a "tip-speed" below 900 feet per minute (4.57 meters per second). Gentle mixing is essential in order to allow the silicone emulsifier molecule to uncoil from a random orientation. The implication is that excessive hydraulic shear can interfere with proper orientation of these large molecules. The slow water transfer under low-shear mixing results in a "crude" emulsion of large water droplets suspended in the "open" structure of the oil phase.

"Slow" water transfer is a relative term that is very dependent on the chemicals involved. Thus slow transfer can mean transferring a water phase, which is normally between 35% and 65% of the batch, into the oil phase over a period of 40 to 220 minutes. Another way to help the silicone emulsifier uncoil is to "seed" the oil phase with 5% to 10% of the water phase. The seeding step involves the slow transfer of a small percentage of the water phase into the oil, followed by a mixing period before the slow water transfer is resumed. The primary difficulty with this method is that two transfer pumps may be required to control the rates at the two extreme transfer rates.

In either case, a gentle mixing period follows the water transfer, with the batch sometimes showing a 1,000 to 5,000 centipoise build in viscosity, indicating that it is ready to be finished.

The finishing step involves converting the large water droplets of the "crude" emulsion into fine droplets that make up the internal phase of the W/S product. High-shear mixing is normally needed in this step. It should be applied as a single pass through a high-shear device with the shear applied via an orifice plate, colloid mill, or in-line rotor-stator homogenizer. A drop-in homogenizer can provide sufficient shear, but batch uniformity may produce acceptable test results of the batch with long-term stability issues due to the variation in final droplet size distribution.

Production of water-in-silicone emulsion systems requires as much attention to the "crude" emulsion step as it does to the finishing step. The water transfer time cannot be cut short. Cold (room temperature) emulsion formation eliminates cooling time providing a faster batch cycle time, provided the production equipment can match the shear energy applied in the lab. These are the two keys to successful W/S processing.

j. Liposome Production

Liposome formulation in the cosmetic industry normally utilizes phospholipids and produces either single- or multi-lamellar vesicles. High-pressure homogenization is the main method for liposome processing. There are two processes commonly employed for manufacture. Both methods are used to achieve a uniform-sized single- or multi-lamellar vesicle. The first utilizes a piston/valve homogenizer at an 8,000–10,000 psi (551–689 bar) operating pressure. Production requires four to five passes to achieve a uniform size distribution of the vesicles. Additionally, a temperature reduction step is required between passes to avoid degradation of active materials and destruction of the vesicles. This method produces vesicles in the range of 300–500 nanometers in diameter. The second method uses two product streams which impinge at 20,000–30,000 psi (1333–2000 bar). For specialized applications, pressures up to 60,000 psi (4000 bar) are available. This method also requires 4 to 5 passes, with temperature reduction between passes. It will result in much smaller vesicle sizes, typically 50–200 nanometers.

Non-phospholipid liposomes can also be produced. High pressures are not usually required for their formation. They are formula-specific, temperature sensitive, and may require specific agitation for their formation. Special controls may be required during their production. Typical vesicle sizes are in the 100–500 nanometer range, with process pressures of 200–1000 psig (13–67 bar).

13.1.3.3 WET SYSTEMS—LIQUID-SOLID SYSTEMS

The production of a cosmetic product often involves the incorporation of a powdered solid material into a liquid. The objective may be to dissolve the powder completely (as with true solutions like salts or preservatives in water), to produce a colloidal dispersion of water-swelling particles (as with bentones and other gelling agents), or simply to disperse insoluble materials, such as pigments. To do this efficiently with a wide range of powder particle sizes, surface characteristics, and liquids of varying viscosities, a variety of mixing equipment is available.

Perhaps the easiest of these processes to carry out is the dissolution of a fairly large, smooth-faced solid, such as salt. The initial incorporation of each crystal into the liquid involves the complete replacement of the air-solid surface with a liquid-solid surface. This may be considered to be a three-stage process of adhesion, immersion, and spreading, Figure 13.22. Immersion is complete when the liquid has displaced all the air and the surface of the crystal has been completely wetted by the liquid. A low surface tension results in a low contact angle (between the liquid and solid), which aids this process. This is a result of the production of a positive spreading coefficient wherein not only does the surfactant decrease the surface tension of the liquid but it also reduces the interfacial energy at the liquid-solid interface.

Not all powders used in cosmetics have favorable size and surface characteristics. The majority are of extremely small particle size and highly agglomerated. The agglomerates will have a complex structure with an uneven surface and will be perforated by cavities of irregular shape. The complete wetting of such structures, involving the penetration of liquid into all the crevices and cavities together with the expulsion of air, is much more difficult. It should be noted that penetration into cavities requires a low contact angle but a high surface tension. This is in conflict with conditions for easy wetting.

Even more complex is the immersion of powders, which swell in liquid to form dispersions of colloidal size, since the particles on the outside of each agglomerated mass tend to swell and adhere to each other, retarding penetration of the liquid to the still-dry core.

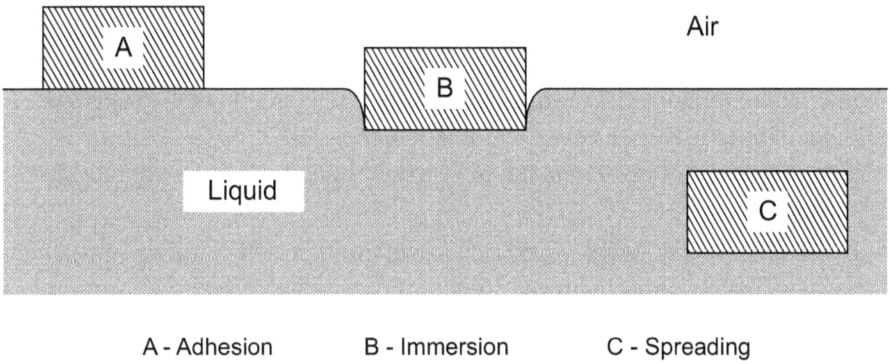

Figure 13.22: Immersion of a solid in a liquid

The forces holding these agglomerates together are precisely the same as those described later in this chapter in the section on powder mixing. The obvious difference, of course, is that these agglomerates are situated in a fluid medium, the physicochemical characteristics of which may enter into the reckoning of bond strength, ease of separation, and likelihood of re-agglomeration. Consequently, the theoretical treatment of particle-particle interaction in liquid media is even more complex than that for dry solids.

In cosmetic processes, the de-agglomeration of solid particles in liquid media can be brought about by a variety of machines. In lipstick processing, for example, pigments are pre-dispersed into castor oil or any other suitable liquid by preparing a coarse mixture that is then processed in a triple roll mill, colloid mill, ball mill, or sand mill. These machines are used specifically because they can deal effectively with high solids content and high viscosities.

For less viscous formulas (e.g., the dispersion of pigments into the aqueous phase of an emulsion), a high-shear device of the rotor-stator type may be used. In this case, ensuring that the whole contents of the vessel are entrained into the shearing head by secondary stirring can shorten processing time. However, the pigments may be externally dispersed, as in the lipsticks mentioned above, before addition to the aqueous phase of the emulsion. Depending on the amount and type of color being used, a rotor-stator type of shearing device may increase the batch processing time.

In view of the fact that a ball mill utilizes only one pass to develop the color (and this may be done outside the manufacturing kettle), it is especially efficient for this method. A wetting agent should be used when dispersing pigments in this manner to aid in de-agglomeration and to minimize re-agglomeration after processing. As with all de-agglomeration, shear stress is critical for the particle disintegration of the agglomerate.

For soluble powders, the enormous increase in the solid-liquid interface brought about by immersion and de-agglomeration ensures that the actual processor dissolution can proceed at the maximum possible rate. For insoluble powders, however, there remains the problem of maintaining a good stable dispersion. De-agglomeration is usually a reversible phenomenon and it can usually be assumed that the opposite process, flocculation (particle accumulation), can take place simultaneously.

In the case of dry powder–powder dispersions, stabilization can be achieved by the introduction of particles of larger size to which disintegrated agglomerates can adhere. In some cases this can be applied to solid-liquid systems, for example, by preextending pigments onto talc before adding them to a liquid foundation base. In many instances all the solid particles might be too small a size for such a process. Under these circumstances, rules similar to those used in emulsion technology can be applied. Thus, some or all of the following means can slow the rate of flocculation:

- The use of surface-active agents (sometimes as polymer coating of the powdered solid) to inhibit flocculation by steric hindrance.
- The manipulation of electrostatic charges on the surfaces of the powder particles.
- The manipulation of the viscosity of the dispersion.

Surface-active agents play a part at two stages in the process of manufacturing a stable dispersion. It has already been seen that the lowering of the solid-liquid contact angle speeds up the wetting process. In practice, the best results are often achieved not with a surfactant, which measurably lowers the surface tension of the liquid, but with what is sometimes described as a surface activator, which reduces the interfacial tension between solid and liquid. These surface activators (which are best described as "dispersing agents") can, if correctly chosen, cause an immediate improvement in the quality of the dispersion, which is manifested by an increase in the color intensity.

The rules for choosing a dispersant are similar to those used for surfactants in emulsions; part of the molecule must have affinity for the liquid medium and part for the solid. A significant difference exists, however, between emulsions in which the two phases have very different chemical affinities) and dispersions of solids in which a hydrophilic solid is dispersed in water. Powders can be processed to coat their surfaces with a chemical (usually a polymer) of suitable characteristics to allow easy wetting and dispersion. Nowhere is this more clearly demonstrated than in the case of water-wettable (hydrophilic) and oil-wettable (hydrophobic) grades of titanium dioxide. In this instance, the same grade of titanium dioxide can be coated with different resins to modify the surface in such a way as to make it wettable by either water or oil. Formulation problems resulting from flocculation are normally resolved before scale-up. Thus, the addition of shear-thinning gums to nail lacquers and of colloidal thickeners to the aqueous phase of emulsions helps to slow down flocculation without materially influencing the basic flocculation process itself. However, reheating of liquid pigmented foundation products sometimes results in unexpected changes of hue, which are often erroneously ascribed to phase-inversion. The truth is that the rate of flocculation of an intrinsically unstable dispersion has been increased because of a drop in viscosity caused by the heating process.

a. Suspension of Solids

If a particulate solid is dispersed in a liquid in which it does not dissolve, if the suspension so formed is allowed to stand undisturbed in a vessel, and if the densities of the two components are dissimilar, some degree of flocculation will eventually take place. Where the particles are present in sufficiently low concentration to have a negligible effect on the viscosity of the suspension, the establishment in the liquid of flow patterns of sufficient turbulence can achieve re-suspension.

The suspension of solids in agitated tanks is frequently encountered in cosmetics processing as an aid to dissolution or as a means of obtaining a good dispersion of particles prior to a change of viscosity of the liquid medium by gelling or cooling. Although the theory concerning flow patterns in agitated tanks has already been discussed, it is necessary to reiterate that it is axial flow that is of prime importance in the movement of solid particles away from the top or bottom of a tank. At the lower viscosities a correctly sized propeller mixer at the correct angle for mixing is the best method for achieving the axial flow. See Figure 13.8 b.

Three conditions can be recognized during the production of a suspension, namely complete suspension, homogeneous suspension, and the formation of bottom or corner fillets [16].

Complete suspension [17, 18, 19, 20, and 21] exists when all particles are in motion and no particle remains stationary on the bottom or surface for more than a short period. Under these conditions, the whole surface of each particle is presented to the fluid, thereby ensuring the maximum area for dissolution or chemical reaction.

Homogeneous suspension exists when the particle concentration and (for a range of sizes) the size distribution are the same throughout the tank. The homogeneous suspension is always more difficult to achieve and to measure than the complete suspension. Nevertheless, homogeneous suspension is very desirable for certain types of cosmetics applications, and particularly so for continuous processing. In practice, for such processes the requirement is only that the particle-size distribution and concentration in the discharge of the homogenizer head and the vessel are the same.

Sometimes heavier particles are allowed to collect in corners or on the bottom of the vessel in relatively stagnant regions to form fillets. This may have the practical advantage of very large savings in power consumption compared with the energy that may be needed to achieve complete suspension (provided, of course, that this saving offsets the loss of the active/solids in the fillets).

In general, it may be said that a propeller at a 45° angle or turbines offer the best advantage for rapid suspension at low power consumption. If, on the other hand, radial-flow agitators need to be used, these should be of relatively large shaft-length to impeller-diameter ratio, be placed close to the bottom of the tank, and have turbine blades extending to the shaft to prevent problems with central stagnant regions.

b. Milling Equipment

There are many products in the cosmetics industry that require de-agglomeration and particle-size reduction. Lipsticks, concealers, foundations, and mascaras are examples. They have high solids content and are composed of pigments, fillers, and other powders dispersed in a liquid base. It is often necessary to reduce the gritty feel that these powders impart on the skin as well as to maximize the color development of the pigmented phases. By taking the portion of the formula containing the oversized and agglomerated solids, one can mill it to wet out and develop the ingredients. A pigmented phase should be milled until the shade cannot be developed further and the grit cannot be detected by touch. The method of milling will determine the required viscosity of the slurry to be processed. Colloid mills, ball mills, and three-roll mills are used extensively to de-agglomerate, and to produce the required feel and shade development. The colloid mill requires the lowest viscosity slurry of the three mill types mentioned and the three-roll mill requires the highest viscosity slurry.

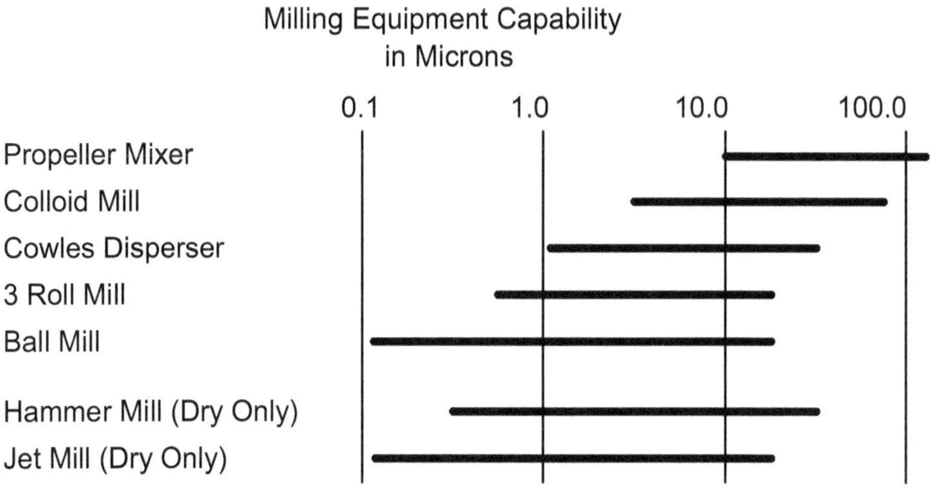

Figure 13.23: Particle-size comparison for milling equipment (some processing may require multiple passes)

c. Colloid Mills

Colloid mills are used as in-line devices. They work by hydraulic shear. The energy they produce is imparted to the product in a thin film. Colloid mills can be used to de-agglomerate pigments or to disperse solids in liquid phases through recirculation. They can be used to build final viscosity in an emulsion system, as a continuous device.

The colloid mill consists of a rotor, a rapidly rotating conical member, which may be smooth, toothed, or grooved, and a similarly machined stator into which the rotor fits. Product is pumped through the mill inlet, and the fluid mixture is forced through the small clearance [ranging from 0.004" (0.1mm) to 0.040" (1.0mm) gap size] between the rotating rotor and stator. The gap size can theoretically be set to 0.001" (0.025mm); however, 0.004" is typically used as a minimum to allow for tolerances due to wear in the rotor and stator. Figure 13.24 illustrates a typical design.

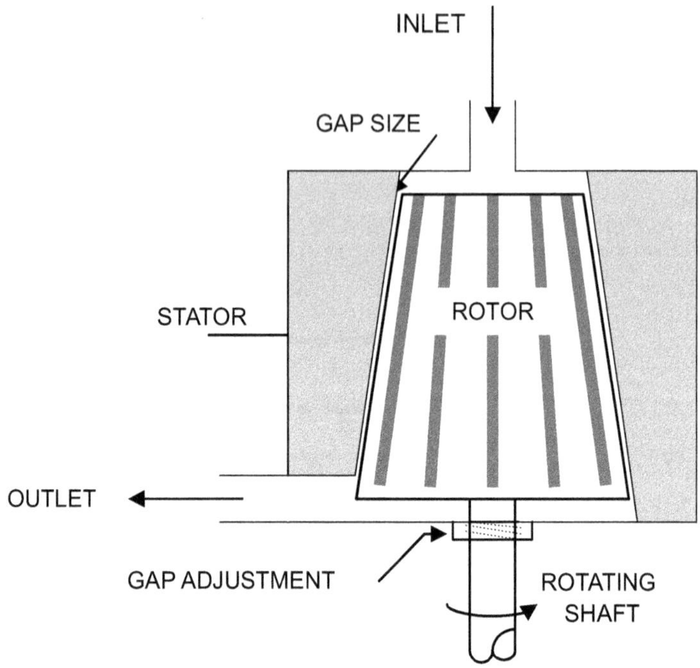

Figure 13.24: Colloid mill

There are three important process variables that affect product output: retention time, tip speed, and gap size. Each of these is a known quantity or can be measured, and each can be adjusted to give the desired result.

Retention time is the amount of time the product is exposed to the milling energy. The longer the product is in the mill, the smaller the particle size will be. Retention time is dependent on the flow rate, rotor speed, backpressure, and the gap size. The flow rate is easily measurable and should be controlled by a positive displacement pump. When rotor speed, backpressure, and gap size are kept constant, flow rate is the only variable controlling retention time. Average tip speed, the linear velocity averaged across the surface of the rotor, is the shaft speed multiplied by the average rotor circumference. Increasing the tip speed imparts more energy to reduce the particle size. Likewise, lowering the tip speed imparts less energy, which lowers particle-size reduction. By varying the gap size, the product is forced through a different opening and a different void volume in the mill. Equation 13.8

Colloid mills are effective tools for reducing the size of particulates and dispersing agglomerates. They are usually scalable from laboratory to production sizes if the style, retention time, tip speed, backpressure, and gap size are all kept constant.

d. Ball Mills

Ball mills are typically used as a side batching or in-process device. Unlike the colloid mill, they are not normally used on the finished product, just the pigmented sub-phase. Ball mills are used extensively in the de-agglomeration of solids (up to 60% concentration for some pigments) into a liquid medium and development of the pigment shades.

The rapid movement of grinding elements (media), which take the form of pebbles, balls, or finer sand-like particles, 1 millimeter or less in diameter, results in the breakdown of agglomerates. The mill style may be horizontal or vertical in which a rotating agitator (rotor) causes the grinding media to rapidly collide. The powder particles to be milled are subjected to both impact and high shear. Heat energy is produced during the milling process, so the milling chamber should be jacketed for controlled cooling. This will protect the product from reaching an unsuitable temperature. Figures 13.25 and 13.26 illustrate the design of vertical and horizontal ball mills. The annular gap or screen is used to retain the media in the mill and allow the milled product out. The milled product or phase may have to be filtered to ensure that any broken or worn media is removed.

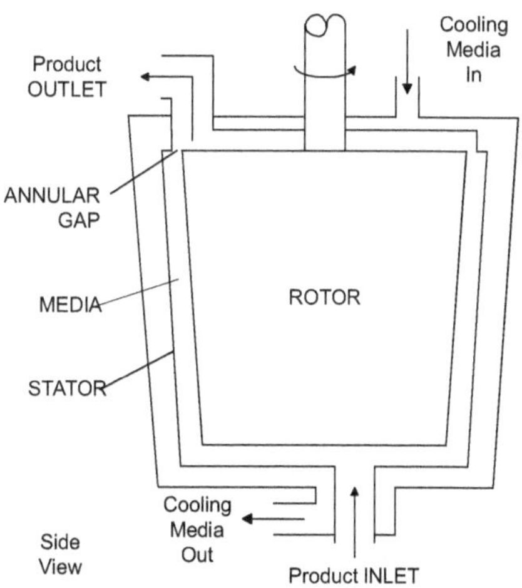

Figure 13.25: Vertical ball mill

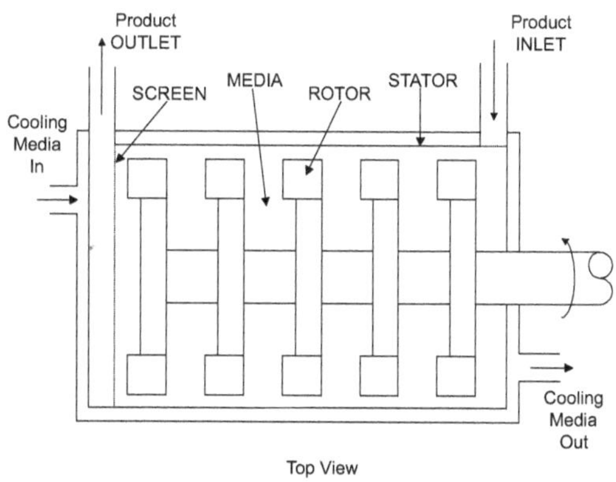

Figure 13.26: Horizontal ball mill

Before a sub-phase can be ball-milled, the powders and pigments first must be pre-dispersed; the quality of this pre-dispersion may affect the quality of the finished grind. It is typical to design the process to have a ratio between in-feed particle diameter to media diameter of 10 and 20 to 1. For example, if the in-feed particles are between 50 and 100 microns in diameter, the milling media should be 1.0 millimeters in diameter [22]. If the media diameter to pre-dispersion phase diameter is not matched, problems may occur. If the particles in the phase are too large, they will enter the ball mill and plug the screen or gap. Although no oversized material will exit the mill, no material will be processed. If the media is too large, particles of the phase will pass between the media and not be efficiently milled. If the size of the media is too small, the power required will be higher and the particle-size distribution exiting the mill will be wider than expected. Some particles will be exposed to high energy as they are processed through the mill, while some will see less as they travel a different route through the mill.

Choosing the proper media size can help control the finished distribution. There are five important process parameters that affect the milled product: retention time, rotor tip speed, media type, media size, and media loading. Each of these is a known quantity or can be measured, and each can be adjusted to give the desired result.

Retention time is the average amount of time each particle is in the milling chamber. Generally, the longer a particle is exposed to the milling energy, the smaller the particle size will be. Retention time is a function of the void volume in the mill chamber and the volumetric flow rate of the slurry. The equations for retention time and related void volume are:

$t = V_v / Q$ and $V_v = V_c - V_m$

Where: t = retention time in minutes

V_v = Void (Available) Volume of the Mill in liters

V_c = Volume of the Empty Mill Chamber, with the Rotor in-place, in liters

V_m = Volume of the Media in the Mill in liters

Q = Volumetric Flow Rate of the Product in liters per minute

Equation 13.8 Mill retention time`

The void volume is a function of the media loading (quantity and size used for the process). As the media loading (V_m) increases, the void volume (V_v) decreases, decreasing the retention time for constant flow. The void volume parameter (V_v) is easily controlled before processing. The flow rate is easily measurable and can be controlled by varying the speed of the product supply pump. Slower flow rates will produce higher retention times, generate an increase in the number of collisions, and yield a smaller particle size. The rotor speed controls the movement of the media, which controls the collision energy imparted to the slurry. Greater shaft speeds generate more collisions, which helps to reduce the particle size.

Choosing the proper media is crucial in getting the desired end product. Size and composition are the important factors. The media diameter must be greater than the annular gap size; otherwise media will be found in the product and normally is at least three to one media diameter to gap. Common media types used are sand, stainless steel, glass, zirconium oxide, and zirconium silicate. The hardness (or density) of the media will determine adequate grinding versus wear on the chamber. Harder (or denser) media will reduce particles better than less dense ones. However, the interior of the mill may become pitted and wear faster. Media which is too brittle may fracture and be found in the product. The breakage pattern of the media (e.g., pulverization, crumbling, or slivers) should ensure that no long slivers or damaged media are passed through the screen and are found in the finished product. Ball mills are widely used in the cosmetics industry today. They are effective tools for grinding and reducing agglomerates. They are usually scalable from laboratory to production sizes if the equipment style, retention time, rotor tip speed, media type, media size, and loading are kept constant.

e. Three-Roll Mills

Three-roll (roller) mills are typically used as side batching or in-process devices. Like the ball mill, they are not normally used on the finished product, just on the pigmented sub-phase. Unlike the ball mill, particles are ground down to reduce their agglomerate size. Roller mills are used extensively in the dispersion of high solids content (and high-viscosity) pigments into liquid media and for full development of the pigment. Typical solids content for a roller mill grind is 50% or higher.

The roller mill consists of three rolls each operating at different speeds and a takeoff knife or doctor blade. The mill reduces particle size by using shear (adjacent rolls operating at different speeds) and mechanical pressure. The first roll (the roll nearest the operator) operates at the slowest speed, the middle roll is faster, and the third roll is the fastest. Material is transferred from roll 1 to roll 2 to roll 3 where it is scraped from roll 3 with a knife-edge blade. In order for the material to move from one roll to the next efficiently, it is necessary for the material being ground to have some tack. Without tack, material transfers very slowly, if at all; but if the material is too tacky, it may pass through the mill too quickly.

The percent solids content of the slurry should be adjusted based upon how well it performs on the roller mill. This needs to be developed in the laboratory. The slurry should be observed at several different points in the process, both in the laboratory and during manufacture.

Production size three-roll mills are manufactured with a slight crown (outward curve) to each roll. This is done so that as pressure is applied the rolls will flatten. The material coming off the knife blade is referred to as the tongue. If not enough roll pressure is applied, the tongue will be longer in the middle and shorter on the ends as seen in Figure 13.27 a. If too much pressure is used, the tongue will be longer at the ends of the roll and shorter in the middle, as seen in Figure 13.27 b. With the proper pressure, the tongue will be even all the way across the knife blade/tongue onto the takeoff plate as seen in Figure 13.27 c.

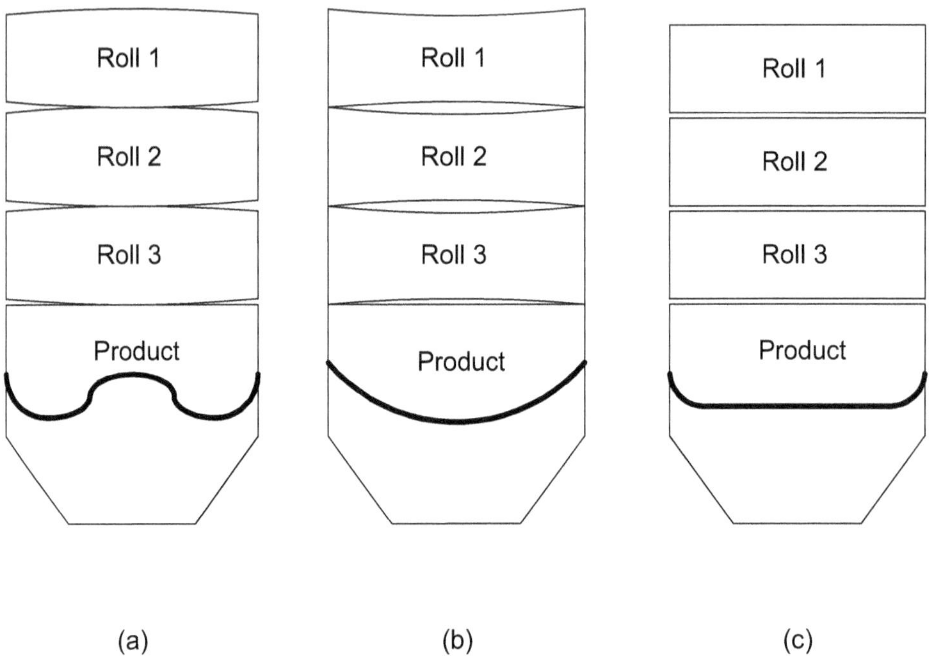

Figure 13.27: Three-Roll mill pressure control

Three-roll mill procedures are time consuming; however, the mechanical energy imparted to the product is very effective. Due to general safety and cleaning difficulties, three-roll mills are not preferred for production. Due to the design of the feed system, particularly during the cleaning operation, items can be drawn into the gaps, called "nips," which pose a safety hazard to the operator. As the rolls are worn, minute pitting occurs. These pits can hold fine pigments and lead to contamination problems with subsequent batches. This enhances cleaning difficulties. Fortunately, based upon the availability of raw materials, it is usually de-agglomeration not particle-size reduction that is required, so alternate systems can be considered.

13.1.4 FILLING

Most cosmetics are filled from stored bulk in machines specifically designed to handle the packaging units of a particular product. Great care must be taken in choosing and setting up these machines. The main problems are due to the limitations of the machines themselves rather than the product being filled. There are at least two areas, however, where a special understanding of production filling requirements and constraints, and formula characteristics are essential for achieving efficient production. These are the molding processes (lipsticks, wax-based sticks, and alcohol-stearate gels—discussed under warm and hot fills below), and compression processes (compressed eye shadow, blushers, and face powders—discussed under filling pressed powder, later in the chapter).

Different products require different types of equipment to be filled effectively, which result in low cost per unit, high filling rates, low maintenance of the systems, and controlled product characteristics. When selecting the proper equipment, two key questions must be answered:

- What are the physical characteristics of the product to be filled—viscosity, flowability, temperature, shear sensitivity, potential for aeration, etc.
- What type of container is being filled—bottle, jar, tube, godet, etc.

The answers to these questions along with (to a lesser degree) the speed at which the product needs to be filled, will determine the type of filler that will be needed. Products are to be handled and transferred from their storage container to the appropriate filling equipment in a clean environment. Cosmetic GMPs are to be practiced and maintained. All equipment must be properly cleaned and sanitized prior to use.

a. Filling Parameters:

There are number of parameters associated with filling that directly impact the aesthetics and quality of the filled cosmetic products. These parameters are:

Type of filling equipment

Temperature of the product at fill

Mixing & shearing of the product just prior to and at fill

Filling speed—velocity through the nozzle

Nozzle size—inlet and outlet diameter, sometimes length

Viscosity & flowability of the product

Specific Gravity

Cooling rate (if filled at an elevated temperature)

Container type and fill opening

b. Filling Machines:

The three types of equipment used for the filling of cosmetics can categorized as follows:

(1) **Positive Displacement Piston filler**—This type of filler is used in many applications across the cosmetic industry. It is capable of handling products with varied viscosity, fluid consistency, and pressure application. It is regularly used to fill products that are of medium to high viscosity. The filler is very accurate achieving consistent fill and is suitable for attaining and maintaining weight claims.

This filler uses reciprocating motion causing fluid to move from one location to another within the unit by way of the rotary valve. The rotary valves ensure that the product moves in one direction while the entrapped fixed portion of the product moves from pump suction to the discharge or dispensing nozzle. The rate of a product's flow inside the piston is proportional to speed of dispensing.

Products such as hot-pour foundations, creams, lotions, viscose lip products (gels and glosses), and mascaras are generally filled using this technology. An example is shown in Figure 13.29.

(2) **Gear Pump filler**—Gear pumps are versatile, operate consistently in either flow direction, and give a constant and even discharge regardless of pressure fluctuations due to supply level changes. It consists of two gears that generate suction on one side and drive the product out to the dispensing nozzle. This filler is often designed to recirculate the product and is normally used to handle products easily deaerated. It can help to control product variability when a weight claim is hard to achieve, particularly if solids can easily settle out (for thin products that contain pearls and pigments to keep the powders suspended during dispensing). A less accurate weight claim is associated with products that need recirculation during fill. The fill is often based upon a timing cycle—product circulates, then fills, then circulates. This filler is used for products that are less viscous, and flow easily such as lotions, and liquid make up. These fillers should not use a gravity hopper since the flow rate will change as the product level changes during the fill.

(3) **Vacuum/Pressure filler**—In vacuum/pressure equipment, the product is either pushed via a pump or gravity system, or pulled via a vacuum system to the container. When the fill reaches the set height, any additional product (overfill) is directed away from the package through a return port incorporated in the filling nozzle, Figure 13.28. The vacuum is used to draw the product into the container to a set height. In these systems, product continually flows through the nozzle, bypassing the nozzle outlet when it is

not filling. Both the excess fill and the bypassed product are returned to the filling hopper. The product is then available to be reused during the filling run. A level sensing system may use a slight air pressure flow that is delivered through a control line attached to the tip of the filling nozzle. A control sensor notes the change in backpressure once product has filled the package and reached the sensing tip of the control line. The sensor then stops the delivery of product to the filling nozzle.

(4) Both types of Vacuum / Pressure / Fill-to-Level filling systems fill to a set level, regardless of the container size, shape, or capacity (internal dimensions of the package). They allow a great deal of volumetric variation while delivering an aesthetic look to the fill. This may be of critical importance for some package designs. The production of plastic packages is much better controlled, dimensionally, than for glass packages. The variation on a glass package volume can be as high as 10% and still be considered acceptable.

A **tube filler** is another form of positive displacement piston filler that is generally used for filling both low- and high-viscosity products such as creams, lotions, gels, conditioners, cleansers, lip balms, and toothpastes. The tube filling machines are equipped with hot-air or hot-element sealing jaws and are configurable to seal the plastic or laminated metal tubes by using automated heating and crimping (press) after dispensing is completed. Metal tubes are crimped using multiple sets of jaws to fold over the tube ends in various patterns.

c. Filling – Low-Viscosity Products (Lotions, Toners, Liquid Makeups)

Vacuum / Pressure / Fill-to-Level equipment can take advantage of the flowability of low-viscosity products to produce a very efficient fill. See Figure 13.28. Low-viscosity products can aerate, foam, and striate during the handling and filling operations and directly affect the esthetics of the fill by producing under fills, wet packages, poor seals, low production yields, etc. Shear-sensitive products raise special concerns when setting up and operating the filling system. Poor setup will result in high recycle and bypass rates, which will continually add shear to the product, and increase the probability of aeration and the potential for contamination. Foam in the filling hopper will probably be produced. By choosing an improper pump type (centrifugal versus positive displacement) and size or misadjusting the vacuum level, significant shear on the product can result. Nozzle sizing is often determined by the constraints of the package. Small nozzle size, along with high production rates, may not work well together. The rates may have to be slowed when small nozzles are used to control the flow near the top of the bottle and limit the shear on the product. These factors can all limit the production rates, and are all key production concerns when any new formula is produced. For efficient production and improved control, low-viscosity products depend on check valves fitted into the nozzles.

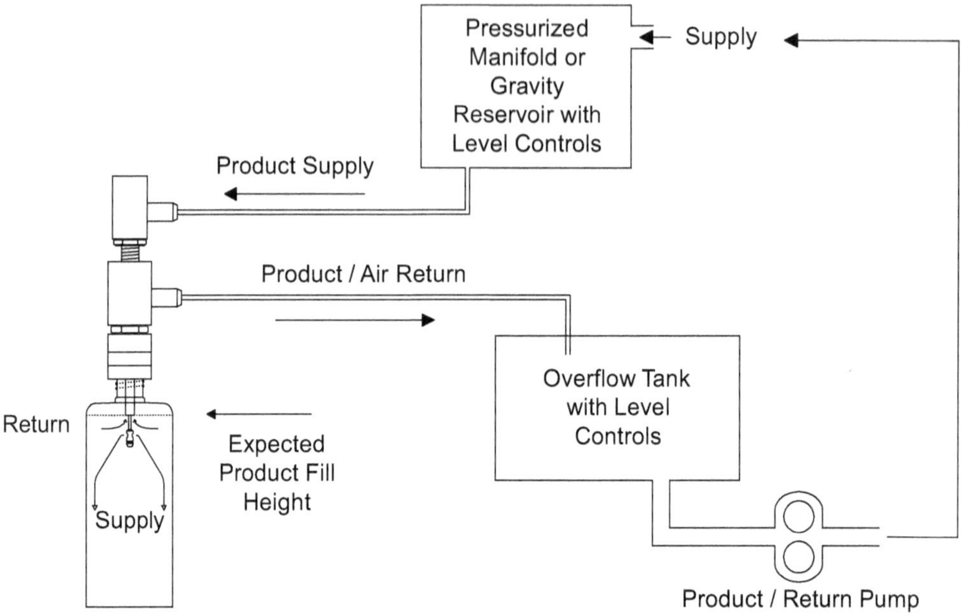

Figure 13.28: Liquid fill-to-level system

d. Filling – High-Viscosity Products (Creams, Mascaras, Masks)

Products in this category will not flow readily without the assistance of an outside force. A Positive Displacement (PD) filler system is required. A PD system includes a controlled pump that works in tandem with a piston or related device, which can overcome friction and flow problems to move finished product through the filler, Figure 13.29. With very viscous products, a pressure hopper and/or ram pump is also needed to supply nonaerated mass to the filling chamber (aerated mass will produce inconsistent fills). The ram pump system contains a plate that lowers into the container as the product is filled. The pump pressurizes the supply container and minimizes aeration as the product is filled. Pressure is often required to maintain product flow to the filling nozzle. A crowder may also be designed into the hopper for this purpose. It is designed to push the mass toward the nozzle slowly while maintaining an air-free environment.

A piston, or positive displacement pump, is then used to dispense the product in a controlled manner. By design, these fillers dispense a reproducible quantity of product for each rotation of the chamber (piston cylinder or pump head). To dispense different quantities, the piston stroke length or the number of revolutions of the pump can be adjusted. High-viscosity products will typically "break off" cleanly from the nozzle tip. Special nozzles are rarely required except to control the curl, or wave, that can be developed upon completion of the fill (ice cream curl).

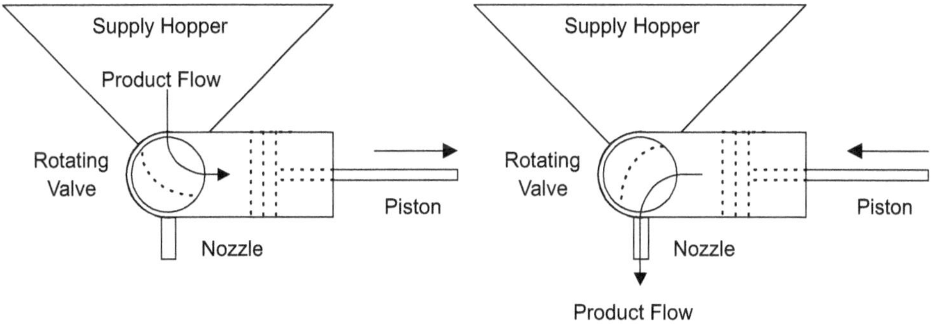

Figure 13.29: Positive displacement filler

Mascaras and masks are generally filled at room temperature. Agitation inside the filling hopper or holding drum is not recommended or required during the filling process (high potential for aeration).

The filling/dispensing speed should be carefully adjusted based upon the flow characteristics of the product. Too fast a rate may create air at the discharge point. A void can be created inside the package, which may affect the fill weight, product aesthetics, and possibly the long-term stability of the product. The nozzle size is determined by the vial or component size, desired fill-weight and shear sensitivity of the mascara—typically as large a diameter as can fit into the package while still allowing air to escape during the fill. For mascara development, it may become very important to know early if the vial's wiper will be received placed in the package. This will force a smaller nozzle to be used, which may shear the product unacceptably.

A product's specific gravity (SG) is critical in determining the minimum/maximum fill weight within a container. Even though the fill weight may be satisfied, aesthetic requirements may not be met (particularly important when the package is clear). For example; a 10-gram fill within a vial may be an issue for a shaded product line—if the product has an SG of 1.0 for a red product and an SG of 0.975 for a blue product, the red shade may fill acceptably while the blue one may be overfilled and have an under-label weight of 9.99 grams.

Troubleshooting for aesthetic and texture: Parameters to look for and address during the filling process are aeration, voids, fill weight, and micro.

Beyond the use of special nozzles, high-viscosity products may require special handling procedures to fill the package without voids. Bottom-up fill capabilities are often required. This also allows a minimum of residual product to remain on the nozzle tip, possibly affecting the fill of the next package. In bottom-up filling, the nozzle will dive down to the bottom of the package and rise as the level of product increases in the package. The timing between the rate of the nozzle rise and the product flow rate must be mated for consistent fill. Sometimes the rates may be stepped instead of continuously controlled to ensure that product flows into all the lower corners of the package. Some difficult-to-fill packages may even require the finished package to be spun to induce the product to move into all of the corners of the package. The packaging of viscous products in clear containers without visible voids is difficult to achieve consistently even with the current state-of-the-art controls and should be avoided. The use of opaque bands on the package to hide potential areas of voids may make the filling operation appear more successful.

Some products will be packaged with a disc placed between the top of the jar and the cap. The purpose of the disc is usually to minimize the air contact with the product in the filled package. This may be due to the activity of the raw materials in the formula, and to the microbiological sensitivity of the product. Other functions of the disc are to minimize a separation of the product at the surface, or to prevent moisture from accumulating after a warm (above room temperature) fill. The determination of proper and acceptable disc contact are troublesome specifications for the line operator and mechanic. One hundred percent coverage is preferred. However, any overfill of the package would mean the disc no longer fits and that product will be squeezed out of the package into the threads. Significant underfill may mean no disc contact at all. Typical contact is between 50% and 80%. The design of the package and the filling system used will determine the actual range. It is typical to produce a bottom-up fill with the ice cream peak for improved contact. The peak is pressed down when the disc is placed, ensuring contact.

Products of low viscosity typically flow easily; they do not require the use of a PD system. PD systems are not as production efficient (they are relatively slow) when compared with the alternate systems described, which can provide higher production rates with fewer problems. However, most low-viscosity products can be filled on the same equipment as used for high-viscosity products (which is often done in the laboratory or pilot plant). Since low-viscosity products typically need check valves fitted into the nozzles, this may slow the filling rate further.

e. Filling—Traditional Lotion Products

Positive displacement pump technology is used for filling lotion products. The product is pulled from the holding hopper by a piston into an entrapped area and pushed to the discharge area to be dispensed. This filler is particularly suitable to use for emulsions because it performs controlled shear to the product during dispensing.

Filling the emulsions does not normally require heating. Most creams are filled at room temperature. However, there are creams that do require a minimum amount of heat (up to 40°C maximum.) in order to flow and allow circulation in the filling system for the ease of dispensing and to meet aesthetic requirement. Hot fill of emulsions will be discussed in a different section.

Creams and lotions that required cold fill (room temperature) normally do not need mixing inside the filling hopper. However, if heating/warming is involved then sweep mixing inside the holding tank is required to ensure product uniformity. It should be noted that the holding tank must be covered at all times to prevent volatile loss (typically water). Most emulsions are sensitive to mixing; therefore the agitation speed must be carefully adjusted to control shearing and prevent separation of the product.

Adjusting and control of the dispensing speed is particularly important as faster speed can increase the shear to the product at the filling nozzle. It may also create air bubbles and leave dispensing mark on the surface of the filled component and therefore affect the aesthetic.

Troubleshooting for aesthetic and texture: examine aeration (SG) and voids. If the product is low in specific gravity, adjust hopper pressure, hopper minimum and maximum loading (head pressure), minimize the distance between product supply container/tank and hopper, check/adjust the nozzle dispensing rate/speed, and adjust and check loose fittings and hoses. Voids may be corrected by checking the nozzle for nicks and bends. Check the product specifications (aged product may form air pockets during storage, adjust dispensing speed (less swirl in the package), and adjust line speed.

f. Filling – Shear-Sensitive Products

The package will have a direct effect on the minimal shear that is added to the product during filling. Typically, a large-diameter filling nozzle will produce less shear on the product during filling than a smaller size. A tube usually has a large opening by design. Therefore, the mass is rarely sheared during filling. Most bottles have a limiting neck size, but plastic is usually larger than glass for the same size cap. Jars may allow the most flexibility but can be a major problem if small promotional pieces are to be handled.

For shear-sensitive products, the pump used to supply the filler as well as whether or not to allow recirculation must be examined. Specially designed low-shear pumps, along with careful setup by the operator can minimize recirculation and control the quantity of shear that may adversely affect the finished product. The limited available adjustments on the equipment may be critical and force some shearing during filling. It may not be possible to maintain all of the "perfect" settings on the systems available to production. The low-shear pumps have special requirements, which can limit their use for normal processing, for example special seal concerns, limited flow rates, and difficulty in cleaning.

g. Filling Shampoos, Conditioners, Cleansers—Products That Aerate

A gear pump filler equipped with diving nozzle is typically used to dispense this type of product. Fill is done at room temperature; these products do not require heating during the filling process. If warming is required for flow, aeration will take place.

The filling speed is critical in filling these types of products. Dispensing speed must be carefully adjusted as it may create unnecessary air or bubbles at the point of dispensing.

Troubleshooting for aesthetic and texture: imperfections to look for and parameters to address during the filling process include aeration and voids. Microbial testing is also important, as most "No Tears" formulas are neutral pH. Every effort must be made to verify air-free bulk is getting to the filling nozzle. To keep from creating voids inside the filled components the appropriate nozzle is required. Controlling dispensing speed and line speed is also important for avoiding air pockets in the tube. These products may be thin enough to allow the air during filling to rise and not affect the products' stability or characteristics, but unless the package is opaque, the fill aesthetics will be poor once the air rises to the surface and the package then looks underfilled.

h. Packaging Lines

Fill-to-level packaging systems lend themselves very well to rotary configurations. A great deal of filling operation is performed within a short period of time. The time can be increased, with a minimal loss of productivity, by increasing the size of the filling circle instead of expanding the entire filling line. With a rotary table, a small increase in table diameter translates to a large increase in available time for the filling process. Therefore, the flow rate can be reduced. Rotary fillers are also used to minimize floor space required for large production runs. Different filling actions can be performed in a limited space, around the rotary table, e.g., bottle placement, filling, cap placement, and bottle transfer to the remaining portions of the packaging line.

For large production packages, greater than 16 ounce (473 milliliter), slower lines are often needed to minimize the shear stresses on the finished mass during extended filling times. For these large-size packages, almost any type of filler can be used. Unlike the related smaller packages, the majority of the production time will now be used during the filling cycle, not bottle handling, capping, and labeling. This slow speed line is often set up in a straight line along a wall to maximize the space in the room for other, higher speed, production lines, Figure 13.30. These orphan lines are usually operated with less automation and utilize production personnel as schedules permit.

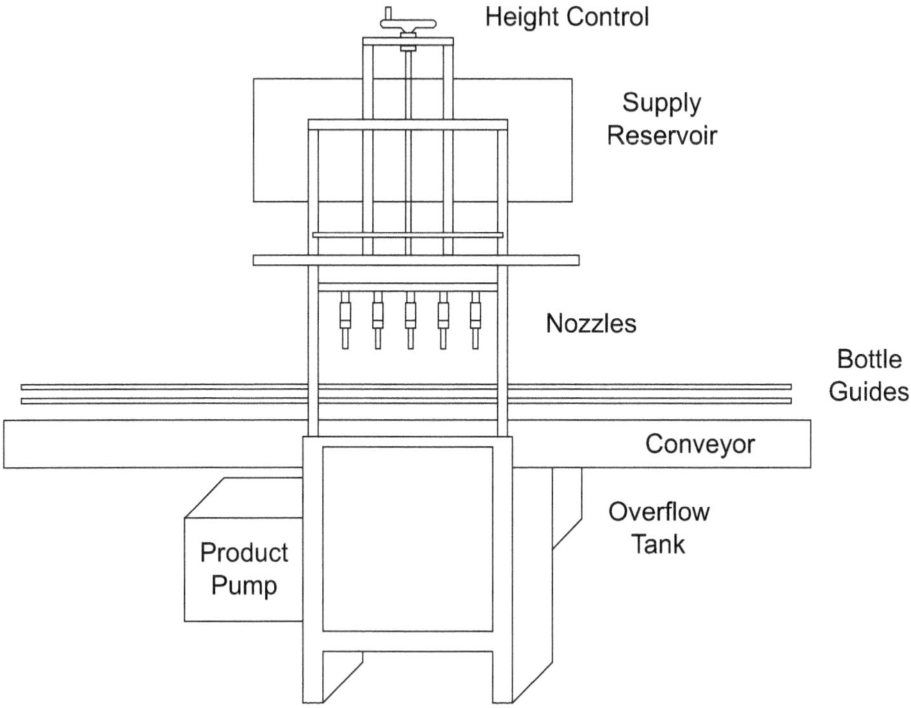

Figure 13.30: Straight Line version of a Rotary Filler

i. Warm and Hot Fills—Creams and Dispersions

Many cream products develop their unique pickup and application aesthetics because the products set up in the package, typically a jar. This requires the fill to be hot (typically 60°C to 80°C). A product that must be filled at an elevated temperature offers a different set of obstacles to overcome. The most important thing to remember is that after bulk manufacture and storage, the product must be heated before filling. This may amount to remanufacturing the product. Most products that require a warm, not hot, fill do not reprocess well and must be filled just after batching. This enforces a Just-In-Time (JIT) operation with its associated production concerns, such as microbiological testing not being completed before filling. Possible concerns include the requirement for warm holding tanks with special agitation, the availability of packaging components, the availability of the production line, and special handling of the finished package.

Moisture is a warm and hot fill problem that is always present and is based upon the formula, package, and filling area. If the product is anhydrous, the only concern is high humidity in the filling area. Moisture from the air in the package's headspace may then condense on the surface of the filled package as the product slowly cools. Droplets of water can easily become locations for significant microbiological growth since it will not combine with the product. Fortunately, this high humidity condition is rarely a concern. If the product contains water, however, moisture can easily collect on the surface during cooling as the water leaves the product at the air interface.

When filling into a tube, this is of minimal concern. The tube is squeezed in use. Any minimal moisture in the headspace will be blended with the product and sheared as it exits the orifice. When filling into a jar, a special cooling operation may be required to minimize moisture on the surface. This cooling operation is time, temperature, and airflow dependent. Its purpose is to cool the filled mass and evaporate any moisture on the surface at the same time. Evaporation is necessary from both an aesthetic and a microbiological standpoint. A disc may be added to the filling process to help keep the available headspace to a minimum and cut down on the time required after filling to seal the package. However, if the amount of disc contact is insufficient, a pool of water may still collect and be the first thing the consumer sees upon opening. A typical cooling tunnel will allow the package to cool for at least twenty minutes with 10°C to 25°C air flowing around and over it. Dust and dirt, as well as microbiological, contamination are concerns during the entire cooling time. A standard protocol should be followed for all fills from the laboratory bench through the pilot plant and into production for consistency and uniformity.

j. Warm and Hot Fills—Godet Products

When a product is not filled at or around the optimum temperature, its hardness or texture may be adversely affected. This is readily noted with the change in payoff or application when filling godets (small pans). Adverse effects can also occur when the product is not remelted to at least the minimum melting temperature. The best way to determine both of these temperatures (reheat minimum and pouring maximum), which may or may not be the same, is to run a heating and cooling curve on a Differential Scanning Calorimeter (DSC). By reading the peaks on the heating curve, one can determine the minimum melting temperature of the highest melting wax. The peaks on the cooling curve indicate at which temperature the waxes will start to crystallize out of solution. Because of solubility factors, waxes will usually crystallize out of solution at a lower temperature than is needed to completely melt them. The optimum filling temperature is usually somewhere above the crystallization temperature and usually, but not always, below the melting point of the highest melting wax.

If a DSC were not available, a rule of thumb would be to remelt the product to a temperature at least as high as the melt point of the highest melting wax in the product. The optimum filling temperature would then become a trial-and-error procedure on the filling line. A good starting point could be determined by pouring a number of pieces at different temperatures in the laboratory.

A key problem for production is in trying to match the aesthetics on the filling line of the "approved" sample, which was carefully poured into the container in the laboratory. A filled product on the manufacturing line may never match the surface appearance of a laboratory-poured sample. This is a particular problem when filling godets. Once the formula is ready for manufacture, a test fill should be performed on the actual filling line or a similar piece of equipment that can be scaled to the actual filling line. This is done to determine true operating parameters and to develop standards that the manufacturing facility can achieve within the expected production rate.

The filling temperature of the product should be the first parameter to be set. The temperature of the product exiting the nozzle is equal or greater in importance than the temperature in the filling kettle. The transfer from the reheat vessel to the filler is done manually or via a transfer pump—follow all local safety considerations (as an example, some facilities do not allow manual transfer above 45°C).

For all hot-pour kettles, the filler must start by purging the product through pistons, transfer hoses, and nozzles. To ensure product uniformity in the filling hopper, both bulk and filled pieces are to be checked within certain time intervals. If the filler is stopped for an extended time, then it must be purged prior to resuming filling into components. When using heated nozzles, make sure the product is not being overheated just prior to filling, particularly if the line is idle. If heat is continuously applied, the section will overheat during the idle times. Unheated nozzles require the mass in the filling kettle to be kept a few degrees warmer than the desired filling temperature in order to provide the correct initial filling temperature. Once the temperature at the nozzle has reached the proper temperature, the kettle temperature may need to be reduced.

Once the correct filling temperature is established, there are other filling parameters that may affect surface appearance and can be set by trial and error. Some of these variables include the nozzle outlet's size and shape. Smaller-size nozzle generally leaves a pouring mark on the surface of the compact. Large-size nozzle may minimize any hot-pour aesthetic filling issues (but may drip onto the transfer belt or the next pan). Tapered nozzle with suck-back capability can facilitate a better fill and minimize most aesthetic issues. Some less complicated nozzle types that may be experimented with are a flared head (outward like a funnel or inward, making a smaller diameter at the tip), a showerhead type (large opening with multiple holes), or a straight-through nozzle. The change in nozzle design can be used to minimize dripping and change the pour dot on the surface of the godet. A moving belt may also shift the pour mark to a location that is aesthetically acceptable. The nozzle's internal diameter and flow rate determine how forcefully the product enters the container. The distance from the filling nozzle to the container affects the spreading of the product into the container.

The different types of container used (steel, aluminum, tin, or plastic) all dissipate heat at different rates, which affects the spreading and cooling rate of the product and often the surface finish. The filling belt speed determines how evenly the product fills the container. It is critical to maintain the temperature, as it can impact the aesthetic and texture of the final product as it flows to the edges of the package. Preheating empty containers just prior to dispensing helps to evenly flow the bulk product to the edges. The purpose of post-heating onto the filled pieces is to even out and smooth the surface of any pour mark, bubbles or pinholes. This applies to all hot-pours. Preheating works particularly well for metal pans. However, if too much heat is applied, the texture of the product may be altered, pearlescent pigments may migrate to the surface, or pigments may settle to the bottom.

The type of conveyor used on the filling line will affect the filling operation—for example, a metal belt will hold heat, while a rubber or fabric belt will not. However, metal belts may be needed for pre- and post-heating. The use of a cooling tunnel for quick cooling of the filled pieces will also affect the finished product's aesthetics. Too quick a set may develop an improper surface appearance or crystalline structure. As stated earlier, a good deal of trial and error is needed to establish filling parameters for a hot-pour product.

Most anhydrous products require constant mixing inside the pre-melt tank and filling hopper. Mixing is required in order to prevent particle settlement or flotation and to avoid burning mass on the vessel's walls, especially when the temperature is elevated. (Heating at most filling lines is done electrically since the plumbing services for steam and condensate are not usually available.) Mixing speed is adjusted based on the texture and quantity inside the vessel to achieve optimum agitation. It must be noted that mixing speed is to be monitored so that no air is introduced to the pre-melt batch inside the kettle before the transfer or filling operations.

Specific gravity (SG) plays a significant role when it comes to filling. Products that are aerated fall outside the specified range and the air bubble or voids can be evident in the filled pieces. If the bulk is found to be aerated, then vacuum must be applied to remove the air from the product.

Two methods can be used to cool the filled products—(1) force-cool; (2) air-cool. Depending upon the nature of the products and test trials performed, it can be determined what type of cooling is needed to achieve the desired aesthetics. Force-cooling is normally done by passing the filled component through a cooling tunnel that has adjustable temperature controller. If air-cooling is desired, longer conveyor belts may be required to allow the mass to cool to a functional temperature to allow handling of the component/package. To maintain aesthetics from formula development into production, the same system must be used to cool the filled pieces. Allowing the pieces to air-cool on a counter for a few hours is rarely reproducible by production. Examine short-term storage in both a refrigerator and a freezer to help develop conditions that can be used by both facilities.

The following aesthetic defects and subsequent corrective actions may improve the end results.

- Pinholes: Adjust mixing speed, filling speed, temperature, angle of heat gun for pre/post-heat, check mass quantity in the vessels, apply vacuum.
- Voids: Adjust preheat, mass temperature, nozzle position and size, determine/adjust appropriate use of diving nozzle, filling speed, adjust angle of heat gun for post- or preheat.
- Discoloration or pearl floatation: Adjust filling temperature, mixing speed, adjust angle of heat gun for post- or preheat.
- Sweating: Adjust line speed, adjust filling temperature.
- Cracking: Adjust filling temperature, temperature in cooling tunnel, adjust post-heat, adjust belt vibration, and handling.
- Pour-marks: Adjust angle of heat gun, adjust nozzle position, filling (dispensing) speed, nozzle size.
- Indentation (dimple): Adjust line speed, adjust cooling temperature, and adjust post-heat.

k. Warm and Hot Fills—Lipsticks, Lip Balms, Suppositories

When filling into a mold (e.g., lipsticks, lip balms, suppositories), key areas of concern are the following: aesthetics, aeration, cooling rate, shrinkage, and finishing steps. The DSC is often used to minimize these issues similar to the godet fills mentioned earlier.

Molds come in two basic designs—book and individual. Book molds contain several sections (leaves) that are held together to allow for filling multiple cavities. These are typically between two and five pieces. The use of the mold allows for complete or partial use of the cavities by the operator. In general, there is a large amount of metal around each cavity to provide good/quick heat transfer. Book molds are usually aluminum, coated/treated aluminum, or stainless steel. Individual molds are built into a filling system. These molds—metal (aluminum, brass, or stainless steel), plastic (used for individual bullets and then discarded or included as part of the package), or a silicone/rubber—are filled and cooled as part of an automatic system's operation. Less metal is involved, so a cooling medium is required to control the product temperature.

All molds may require preheating or warming prior to the fill to aid in flow to the tip/edges. Most book-style molds are filled with an overflow condition. The overflow is removed prior to removal of the bullets. This ensures a complete fill after cooling, which often produces sinkholes at the top (fill end) of the stick. Sinkholes are a result of a contraction of the solidifying product that begins at the cooled surface. The cooling of the mold may take place through a chilled bath (liquid), on a chill-table (metal contact), chill-tunnel (circulating air), or in a refrigerator or freezer (circulating/stagnant air). Variations of these techniques can be duplicated from the laboratory through production. Air-cooling in the laboratory, however, cannot be duplicated in a production facility. Most godets contain very little mass, so production can simply use a longer belt to allow for a longer cooling time, when compared to the laboratory. Cooling time is more important for bullet-shape products that may partially set quickly, but finish developing their crystalline structure after an extended time, which may range from several minutes to 24 hours. This makes immediate handling of the just-molded stick a problem for many production designs. Automated systems may have the ability to perform a second fill to fill-in the sinkhole. New aesthetics should then be examined when compared to the laboratory fill.

"Old-time" lipsticks contained high levels of waxes with castor oil. These sticks would shrink a consistent amount during cooling. This shrinkage allowed for easy removal from the molds and consistent insertion into the components. Newer sticks develop a gel structure, which may not shrink as much. This means it is more difficult to remove from the mold, and components may need to change to ensure functionality. Be aware of the potential issues during development—extra cooling or lower-temperature cooling may minimize the difficulty, if the production facility has the equipment available.

Silicone/rubber molds were developed to minimize this contraction issue associated with many newer formulas. After the filling and cooling cycles, the mold stretches away from the bullet allowing for easy removal and insertion into the component. Decorations are also possible, as the bullet does not slide out of the mold. Cooling rate is however an issue to be examined. Silicone and rubber are natural insulators, so the temperature removal is less efficient than for metal molds.

Lipsticks are normally filled in a mold with the finished tip down. Lip balms are normally filled directly into the case, top up. Other hot-fill products can be produced using variations of these two methods. Sinkholes are sometimes believed to be good for a stick product, assuming they do not interfere with the lift mechanism. They are said to offer two outer surfaces for increased strength. The additional strength is formula related and should be reviewed for every shade of every product produced (rarely done). To minimize aeration of the molded sticks, the mass may have a vacuum applied to it just before filling. This assumes the mass to be liquid and not contain key volatiles that may be removed under vacuum conditions. The quantity of vacuum necessary will be formula and temperature dependent. Improved filling methods can also minimize aeration during fill. These methods include the use of diving nozzles, slanted molds for improved flow into the cavities, and slow flow rates to minimize swirling of the mass as it leaves the nozzle. Most aesthetic defects and subsequent corrective actions for lipsticks are the same as those for godets discussed earlier.

Since the apparent volume of product is different in a stick from a godet, if a softer texture is desired, then a lower fill temperature is used. On the other hand, to achieve a more rigid (harder) stick, higher-temperature fill is often used. Small temperature adjustments are often required to address the normal variations in raw materials over the life of the product. Acceptable ranges should always be "suggested" during the initial transfer from R&D to production. If a significant change is required, R&D should investigate the cause even if the aesthetics are acceptable using the "new" filling temperatures.

Finishing of the sticks is product specific. Most lip balms have a waxy texture that is acceptable to the consumer. Also, the finished package is rarely elevated completely before use. Therefore, a minimum of treatment is required. Lipsticks are not as simple. The consumer will often raise the bullet to near its full height before use; the entire appearance must be acceptable since it is continually in view. A "flaming" operation is usually performed to improve the finished appearance of the sticks. Although a gas flame may be used, alternate heat sources are also used: heat guns (hot-air heating) and lamps (induction and convection heating). The heat is used to melt any mold marks or other imperfections in the lipstick and to produce a smooth, shiny surface appearance. Different production techniques are available ranging from fully automated systems (that include the pouring, molding, insertion into cases, and "flaming") to 100% manual systems. The choice will be dependent upon the formula, the finished package, and the production requirements. Some of the testing and assessment criteria that are done to ensure quality of the lipstick bullet, are to evaluate the hardness, strength, texture, payoff, stick finish/shine, discoloration, bullet alignment/insertion, and pinholes.

l. Antiperspirants and Deodorants

Antiperspirants (A/Ps) and deodorants are processed much like other cream and lotion emulsions using similar equipment and processing methods. High-shear mixing (homogenizer or colloid mill) is used to ensure complete dispersion of the solids, typically the actives, in the formulas. One must remember to follow government regulatory guidelines for A/Ps, which are regulated as "over-the-counter" (OTC) drug items in the United States. Most deodorant sticks contain very low levels of solids, but the filling issues are similar.

Stick formulations offer a filling challenge. Like lipsticks and other hot pours, the filling operation can be more critical than the processing of raw materials into the final formula. For sticks to set properly:

- The mass must be hot enough so that it flows into and around the component elevator.
- The mass must eliminate "white spotting" caused by the batch crystallizing on the case walls.
- Pour marks, typically along the case wall created by hot spots where liquid is ejected from the filler nozzle, must be eliminated. Post–surface treatment is awkward at best.
- The mass must set up quickly without shrinkage. A quick set is needed to prevent the suspended solids from settling and to effect a good surface appearance. Shrinkage produces a poor appearance to the consumer and can affect the package mechanism (the product may shrink away from the mechanism so the package cannot function).

Thus, the formulation must be held just above its drop point with sufficient agitation so that the active ingredients, usually alumina complexes, are kept uniformly suspended while the product is filled. The drop point can be accurately determined using a DSC, or by measuring the temperature at which a solid sample liquefies and "drops" out of a test apparatus. Jacketed hoppers with mixers that are capable of holding mass within ±1°C, heat-traced lines and filler assemblies, preheating of the packaging component(s), and the use of cooling tunnels are normal for stick manufacture. In large-scale operations the mass is often recirculated from a jacketed mixing vessel through a customized filler manifold on a specialized filling line. A number of these filling operations, and the equipment associated with them, have been patented. Because of the complexity, it is advisable to utilize "make-and-fill" or semi-continuous processing for A/P and deodorant sticks. If the filling is separated from the compounding step, it is imperative that measures be taken to ensure that uniform product be delivered to the filler. The bulk can easily striate as it sets up in storage. The solid bulk must be sliced vertically for proper remelting, or the entire contents of each storage container completely melted and mixed to uniformity before it is brought to filling temperature.

13.1.5 SCALE-UP

The cosmetics industry has been considered collateral to the fashion industry. The driving force for the product development efforts of both industries is the marketplace. The cosmetic chemist is faced with the challenge of formulating products with active ingredients, rheology, and aesthetic characteristics dictated by the marketing group. Laboratory-scale equipment is used to develop and achieve the desired product characteristics. The chemist's beaker is the place where the scaling process begins, which will culminate in production's vessels. It is common to develop a process that fits current manufacturing equipment because the time to launch a new product is almost always short and the lead-time to purchase and install new equipment is almost always long.

It is not unusual for a product that was successfully developed in the laboratory to exhibit quite different characteristics when it is transferred to production. As the product is transferred from a small, laboratory-scale apparatus to large-scale production equipment, a difference in conditions is experienced. Even if a pilot plant is available for an intermediate scale, there is no guarantee that problems will not be encountered during manufacture of full-scale production batches. Scale-up, which is of fundamental importance to the efficient manufacture of cosmetics, is an extremely complex subject because the variables that determine the distribution of forces within a processing vessel vary considerably as its size and volume change.[8]

Process scale-up is typically an engineering function, and this chapter is written to provide information to the formulator that would not ordinarily be available. In general, the formulator will develop a product without sufficient awareness of the problems that can arise during scale-up (other than raw material variations from the vendors). The pilot plant is then an essential and valuable tool in choosing the equipment and processes needed for full-scale production. This is an area where a fundamental understanding of unit operations and a willingness to experiment proves most fruitful.

The items most often considered by the process team during scale-up from the laboratory bench to production are:

- Mixing

  Impeller dimensions and types (e.g., 1.5 pitch marine style, 316 stainless steel)

  Impeller tip speed (e.g., RPM and diameter)

  Impeller diameter to tank diameter (D/T ratio)

  Turnover rate (number of batch turnovers per unit time)

  Flow profile (based upon the impeller and vessel configuration and batch loading)

- Heat Transfer

  Heat transfer medium

  Heating and cooling rates

  Maximum and minimum temperatures (batch and vessel walls)

- Mass Transfer

  Phase transfer rates

The task of the process team is to understand which characteristics are controlling the process, which ones must be kept constant, and which may be allowed to vary.

One method of scale-up is to develop the product on the bench using plant (full-scale) limitations. In this method, mixing times, heating/cooling rates, and phase addition times will be held constant from the laboratory to the pilot plant, and into full-scale production. The disadvantage of this method is that it will stifle creativity at the bench due to current manufacturing limitations. The existing plant becomes the model, and even the pilot plant will be designed to mimic its environment and limitations. If a cosmetic company is to prosper, it must continue to expand its technology base with new and innovative products and up-to-date production equipment in which to make them. Basing all scale-up on the plant will not lead to the degree of innovation necessary to achieve vigorous corporate growth. A more progressive approach to the scaling process makes newer technology accessible to the chemist through the pilot plant and the processing team. The formulator now has the resources of a process team to not only guide a new product from bench to production, but to suggest and institute new technology to improve the entire process. In this approach, the formulating chemist and process team will drive the development effort forward so that the manufacturing plant will purchase and install new technology to manufacture new products.

a. Agitation

There are many different types of mixers used in the cosmetic industry. The marine propeller works well at viscosities below approximately 5000 centipoise. Above this viscosity paddle-type mixing is usually required. For improved reliability, three rules to apply during scale-up are:

- The same design propeller should be used in the laboratory, pilot plant, and in manufacturing.
- The mixer tip speeds (linear velocity) should be maintained within the same magnitude.
- The batch turnover rate should remain constant.

The batch turnover rate is calculated using the pumping data supplied by the propeller manufacturer. The liters per revolution (or gallons per revolution) data supplied are usually based upon water as the medium being mixed. As stated earlier, the mixing time required to ensure that every part of the mixture has passed through the mixing impeller at least once, is for three times the theoretical flow rate.

The scale-up team needs to be aware that propeller mixers used in the laboratory are drastically oversized. Increasing the diameter or speed of the mixing blade will increase the horsepower requirement throughout scale-up. Increasing the blade diameter has a much greater effect on horsepower than increasing speed. To maintain scalability from the laboratory through production, a standard D/T and tip speed should be used. This will cause the most difficulty for the formulating chemist since the movement in a 1-kg beaker will appear to be minimal. It is the job of the Process Team to understand this limitation and adjust to a scalable impeller when the product enters the Pilot area.

b. High-Shear Mixing

High-shear mixing typically refers to the use of a homogenizer. There are many homogenizers on the market. As with propeller mixers, their characteristics need to be determined and understood before use. Unfortunately, the data available through the manufacturer is often minimal and may not relate to the formula under development. Data developed by the manufacturer most often were gathered using water as the working fluid (or the data may be based upon a single formula from another industry, typically pharmaceuticals). Actual data must be developed for each process and refined for each formula. To make scale-up easier, the shear developed over time must be quantified. The change in viscosity over time and/or particle-size reduction over time data are required.

The same types of problems exist with homogenizers as with propeller mixers: homogenizer speed, peripheral speed, homogenizer diameter to tank diameter (D/T ratio), turnover rate (flow per unit volume), homogenizer diameter, and flow profile. As with propeller mixers, the equipment used in the laboratory is usually oversized. In-line homogenizers allow for additional control and can make the scale-up process easier, but may require very long process times. Drop-in homogenizers are more difficult to scale-up since additional agitation is required to help ensure all particles or dispersions are passed through the homogenizer.

When scaling products that require rotor/stator homogenizers from the laboratory to production, several major criteria should be addressed. The first consideration is to keep the design of the homogenizer constant whenever possible. Second a constant shear rate should be achieved by maintaining the peripheral (tip) speed of the rotor constant for all batch sizes. Tip speed is defined as the linear velocity of the rotor tip at a given speed, and is calculated as follows:

$$T = (\pi \times D)\ (R)$$

Where T = Rotor Tip Speed in meters per minute

D = Diameter of the Rotor in meters

R = Rotor speed in revolutions per minute

Equation 13.10 Tip Speed

The third consideration should be the flow rate through the homogenizer. By maintaining the batch turnover rate constant for all batch sizes, the shear rate per unit time will be maintained. This ensures that the same shear is imparted to the product over an equal time period (this is to be controlled in the Pilot area as well as throughout production). Additional concerns are homogenizer diameter to tank diameter (D/T ratio), turnover rate (flow per unit volume), and the flow profile.

c. Heat Transfer

When a product has been satisfactorily produced on the bench, the set of parameters used in its manufacture must be duplicated in the production environment. Heat transfer on the bench is controlled most often by a steam table or hot plate for heating, and a water/ice bath for cooling. Agitation is provided in order to ensure the reaction mixture is homogeneous in both temperature and composition. The formulating chemist is very concerned with the batch process temperatures because, in order to form a proper emulsion, the waxy components must be completely melted. Other raw materials have maximum and minimum temperature parameters (to maintain stability and efficacy), which also must be respected. During mixing of the oil and water phases, one must maintain a particular temperature and provide enough agitation to allow the proper formation of the emulsion. The combination of temperature and agitation should ensure the desired results.

What is often not given proper consideration is the heat transfer rate. How fast or slow the product is heated or cooled is often critical to bringing the process successfully from the bench to production. The process team is faced with the problem of duplicating the bench process (small batches, short heat/cool cycles) in production (large batches, slow heat/cool cycles). A one-kilogram batch can be heated from 25°C to 85°C in 20 minutes. This is a three degree-per-minute average rate. This rate is easy to attain in the lab, but is difficult or impossible to attain in production on a 2,000-kg continuous stirred-tank reactor (CSTR). If this average rate must be attained in order to make satisfactory product, the process team will have a difficult time. In order to increase the heating rate, process development and production must raise the steam pressure to attain a higher kettle jacket temperature. This can lead to situations where components of the batch can be burned onto the kettle wall. Active ingredients and preservatives may be overheated, voiding their usefulness in the product. Carbomer and gum solutions may produce flakes on the kettle side, which under side-wiping conditions may result in specks and/or graininess in the final product.

Once a batch is at a high temperature, the time at which it remains there may be critical due to volatile and heat-sensitive raw materials. Fortunately, the heating rate is seldom a scaling problem because its rate is rarely the critical processing factor.

The cooling rate is often more critical than heating rate because of the need to allow waxes and gels to set their structure in the desired manner. If the product is a complex emulsion with an inversion temperature, attaining the proper rate of cooling through this point is absolutely critical. Because the energy-input rate due to mixing must be constant, lengthening the cooling time in production may result in a ruined emulsion due to overmixing (the cooled waxes are now worked more than those in the laboratory, so a different structure develops).

The chemist normally will not use a heat transfer medium other than tap water for cooling. This can range from 10°C to 18°C or more depending on location and season. Ice may be added occasionally, if the product must be quick-cooled. The process team must also attain the same cooling rate upon scale-up. If too fast a cooling rate is demanded, the process team may respond by providing a jacket temperature lower than normally used by the chemist in the laboratory. This may result in freezing or crystallization on the kettle surface. If the product contains many waxes, crystallization may occur prematurely and the final product may be grainy, lumpy, and not meet specifications.

The reason for the variation in time-versus-temperature data when a product is scaled from a beaker in the laboratory to a CSTR in production is the ratio of kettle volume to jacket surface area available for heat transfer. In any CSTR scale-up system, as one goes from a small volume to a large one the volume of material to be heated/cooled increases as a cubic function, whereas the surface area increases as a square function. This exponential difference must be overcome in order to provide the proper heat transfer rate. As a typical illustration of this processing dilemma, a one-kilogram cream or lotion batch may be cooled with tap water at 12°C from 78°C to 30°C in approximately 16 minutes. This is a 3°C per minute average cooling rate. For the same product in a 100-kg kettle, using the same temperature tap water at optimum flow rate, the average cooling rate slips to approximately 1.5°C per minute. If we scale to a 500-kg kettle, this rate is even less favorable. Typical rates can be as low as 0.15°C per minute or less, depending on jacket quality, design, etc. What happens during this additional cooling time as we scale from small to large? Mixing is prolonged, and may not duplicate the product cooled on the bench by the chemist at a rate of 3°C per minute. For this reason, *the chemist must strive to keep laboratory conditions similar to what is attainable in production*. And, where the Chemist cannot maintain the conditions, the Pilot Plant **MUST** maintain them.

Not all products react adversely with bench-to-production variations. There are many products robust enough to withstand all but the most extreme variations. But as the science of cosmetics progresses, emulsion systems for creams and lotions, soap systems for shampoos/conditioners, and gels for body washes are becoming very sophisticated and more sensitive to process variations. Thus, heat transfer and heat/cooling transfer rate should always be considered carefully during formulation and scale-up.

d. Mass Transfer

In scaling up or down, phase addition times should remain constant. It is important that the rate of dilution remain constant as the batch size changes from the laboratory bench to production. This is particularly true for emulsion products during the emulsification steps. Maintaining this requires a conscious effort at the laboratory level. Since production often cannot transfer at rates that the chemist uses at the bench (seconds), without safety being a concern, laboratory processing must be based upon actual production capabilities. Even a slow laboratory transfer may be too fast for production once the rate is scaled. One hundred grams in thirty seconds for a one-kilogram batch is a slow dripping addition. For a 2000-kg production batch this becomes 200kilograms in 30 seconds (with comparable agitation in the vessel). Since the mixing rate is slower, particularly for viscous systems, the dilution and related transfer rate should also be slower. Most emulsions will have a transfer phase of 10–30% of the batch. In the pilot plant and in production, this phase should transfer in 10 to 30 minutes (silicones are a noted exception). *Laboratory operations must allow for similar addition rates.* Since the transfer phase is usually hot, partial additions over the expected time period are better than a slow addition at an uncontrolled temperature.

13.1.6 DRY SYSTEMS

Table 13.1 distinguishes between two types of solid-solid mixing operations: those concerned with segregating powders, and those with nonsegregating or cohesive powders. The essential difference between these two categories relates to the properties of the powders themselves and, in particular, to the freedom with which individual particles have to move independently of their neighbors. Free-flowing powders exhibit many process advantages (such as easy storage, easy flow from hoppers, smooth flow into packages), but have the disadvantage that they tend to segregate unless all the constituent particles are of very similar shape, density, and size. Cohesive powder, on the other hand, lacks mobility and individual particles are bonded together and move as clumps or aggregates. Although segregation is not a problem (except, as can be seen, at very small scales of scrutiny), cohesive powders are difficult to store and do not easily flow from hoppers (see Bulk Powder Storage).

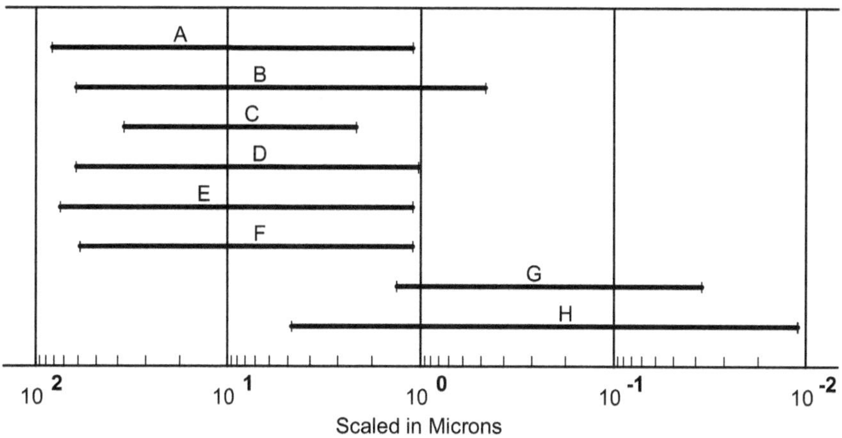

In a powder mass, there are forces at work that tend to make the particles bond to each other and these are balanced by the gravitational mass of the particles, which causes them to fall apart again. Although the bonding forces, for a given powder, are largely independent of particle size, their gravitational mass is not. Since the gravitational forces are based upon the mass of the particles, particles will stick together only when they are small enough for the gravitational forces acting on them to be much smaller than the bonding forces. Powders composed primarily of such particles exhibit cohesive characteristics and those consisting of larger particles tend to be free flowing. To a first approximation, the division between the two types of powder is approximately 50 μm; below this particle size, powders are generally cohesive.

A - Titanium Dioxide	B - Magnesium Carbonate	C - Mica
D - Zinc Stearate	E - Micas coated with Titanium Dioxide	F - Talc
G - Organic Pigments	H - Inorganic Pigments	

Figure 13.33: Range of particle size of some powders used in cosmetics

Figure 13.31 shows the particle size range of commercial grades of some powders commonly used in cosmetics production; by inference, it will be noted that they are all predominantly cohesive in nature.

The nature of the bonding forces between powder particles is of fundamental importance to many industries and is well understood.[23-26] The characteristics of these forces, which are essential to understand, are as follows:

- The forces operate over very short distances. Particles must be brought into very close contact to obtain maximum agglomerate strength (as in pressing).
- The forces are greatly enhanced by the presence of any liquid—particularly if it is easily capable of wetting and spreading over the particle surfaces (like most powder binders).

- The forces that create the agglomerates are very much weaker than those holding the particles themselves together. That is, it is much easier to break up agglomerates than it is to break up a primary particle (most milling is just de-agglomeration, not true particle-size reduction).
- The probability of a small particle bonding to a larger one is much greater than that of a particle bonding to another of the same size.
- Particle shape has as important a relationship to the bonding force as particle size since available surface may determine if particles can get close enough to bond.

a. Blending Equipment

Powder eye-shadows, face powders, and powder blushers are commonly composed of the following types of material:

Talcs	Pigments	Liquid binder systems
Micas	Pearl agents	Preservatives

The order in which these ingredients are processed and the mixing that carries it out are specific to the type and color of product produced.

The completed process is specific to, and depends largely upon, the types of equipment that are used. A satisfactory powder product, when examined under high magnification, is seen to consist of small agglomerates or single particles of the pigments adhering to and covering the surface of the larger talc or mica particles. Improperly processed powders contain larger agglomerates of pigments existing as discrete entities and separate from any talc or mica particles and unevenly coated talc or mica particles. When rubbed, for example between finger and skin surface, such improperly processed powders change hue as these agglomerates are broken and the smaller pigment groups are released and follow their natural tendency to coat the larger particles and the skin. This process is often referred to as the "extension" of pigments onto talc or mica. This "extension" is often intentionally performed separately as an intermediate step in the process. This allows the overall process to flow smoothly while allowing extra processing and testing of the "extension" before use.

The processing of bulk pigmented powder products is dominated by the need to achieve adequate "extension" on an industrial scale. Of all the devices that have from time to time been tried, none has proven more popular than the hammer mill, Figure 13.32.

Since the pre-mix is an additional operation and adds to the processing time and cost, the mixer that is selected must be as efficient as possible. In the past, the most widely used mixer was the "ribbon blender," which comprises a horizontal drum containing a rotating axial shaft that carries ribbon-like blades. In such a device, the pre-mix can take between 20 and 60 minutes. Other mixers are now the standard (V-Mixer and Double Cone), which utilize higher energy input and are quicker to achieve the same level of randomness in the finished mix. Table 13.6 summarizes the properties of some of the more conventional powder mixers. Since it is relatively easy to achieve good mixture quality (at a large scale of scrutiny) in cohesive powders, any mixing device will eventually produce a satisfactory, even distribution of components. This assumes that no dead spots, where mixing does not take place, are present. The dead spots can be "controlled," typically through manual scraping by the operator during processing, if required.

It is typical to add the binder as a liquid after the preliminary mixing stage. Solid waxes may be included in the binder if they are added at a sufficiently elevated temperature to ensure complete liquefaction. The binder may be poured or pressurized through a suitable orifice in the mixer. It is preferred to spray the binder into the mixer cavity as an aerosol through a venturi or similar orifice/ nozzle device. This procedure helps to distribute the liquid more evenly and avoids the formation of wet, lumpy areas in the powder body. Detrimental heat can develop during the manufacture of these high solids formulations. Many times liquid binder sequences (oils, fragrances, preservatives, actives, etc.) are added that must be well mixed to avoid spotting. If they are heat-sensitive or volatile, allowing the blending or milling operation to overheat these components may damage the integrity of the batch. (Most spray nozzles are designed using water. Surface tension of oil binder tends to produce a much poorer quality spray than a water blend. Care must be taken when choosing nozzles, as each binder may behave differently, but production may have limited nozzle capabilities.)

The separation of large agglomerates of powder and binder, which takes place in the milling step that normally follows the binder addition, assures the completion of the wetting process provided the binder is correctly chosen. Should the binder still appear to be unevenly distributed after the passage of the powder through the mill, the product can often be rescued by passing it through as fine a mesh sieve as possible. (Additional milling has its own concerns that are discussed in later sections.) The addition of the binder through high-pressure nozzles improves the fineness of the spray. However, some blending vessels cannot handle the higher pressures, usually 100 to 3000 psig (6 to 200 bar). In general, the finer the liquid addition, the more control of the finished batch is available. An alternate design to the high-pressure spray concept uses cutters to improve the distribution of the liquid and may not require the additional milling step. The cutters provide the additional energy to disperse the binder as smaller droplets in a uniform fashion.

Table 13.6: Conventional Powder Mixers

Type of Mixer	Batch / Continuous	Main Mixing Mechanism*	Speed of Mixing	Process Concerns	Ease of Cleaning	Energy Consumption	Quality of Extension
Horizontal drum	B or C	Diffusive	Poor	Quality of mix	Good	Low	Poor
Löedige/Littleford -type (Plough-shear) (with cutters)	B	Convective	Good	Dead spots at ends	Fair	Medium	Fair/Good
Ribbon Blender	B	Convective	Poor	Dead spots at ends	Fair	Low	Poor
Nauta Mixer (with cutters)	B	Convective	Good	Slow top to bottom blending	Fair	Low	Fair
V-Mixer (with cutters)	B	Diffusive	Fair	Batch size to volume of equipment	Good	Medium	Fair
Airmix	B	Convective	Good	Noisy	Poor	Low	Excellent
Double Cone or CBM** (with cutters)	B	Convective and Diffusive	Excellent	Batch loading	Good	High	Fair
Bowl Granulator (with cutters)	B	Convective and Diffusive	Excellent	Batch loading and scale-up	Good	High	Excellent
Extruder	C	Diffusive	Poor	Formulate to the equipment	Fair	High	Fair
Fluidized Bed	B	Convective and Diffusive	Good	Formulate to the equipment	Fair	High	Poor

B (Batch)—Discrete processing of ingredients

C (Continuous)—Continuous processing of ingredients

* All Mixing Mechanisms include Bulk Flow

Cohesive Mixing: natural or forced combining of particles during blending

Distributive Mixing: controlled or uniform diffusion of particles during blending

** CBM—Containerized Batch Mixing

Batch loading will determine the effectiveness of the mix in any particular vessel. Overloading the processing capacity of a vessel will lower the quality of the mix and possibly increase the temperature during processing. Undersizing the capacity will limit production and affect the quality of the liquid binder distribution. *All scale-up should ensure proper and consistent batch loading throughout—bench, pilot, and production.* For CBM and related higher-energy systems, the loading is between 5 and 8 kilograms per cubic foot (28.3 liters) of vessel contents. Acceptable products can be produced within these ranges. For bowl granulation, the loading is less than 20% of capacity and cannot be varied from vessel size to vessel size.

The use of the liquid binder to assist in the development of color is a technique to be used only under special circumstances. The liquid binder will assist the high-shear equipment to disperse the pigments onto the chosen substrate. However, the pigments will be much more temperature sensitive to color shifting after the liquid has been added. Therefore, each lot of the chosen colors will extend out differently. Extending the pigments and then properly distributing the binder as separate steps can minimize this effect. A special case needs to be considered when dealing with organic pigments. These will darken significantly with heat. Some processes are designed to include this effect. However, a slight hydrogen sulfide odor may be noted when this takes place. Also, the color is not a more intense version of the original shade, but a less vibrant, dirtier, deeper version. To match the shades produced in the laboratory, all development and production must use the same method of extending the pigments along with the same temperature controls.

Pearl agents, especially the titanium-coated micas, present a special problem. Many of these brittle materials, which depend on their size to achieve the desired effect, are prone to disintegration in the hammer mill. For this reason, they usually have to be mixed into the bulk after its passage through the mill, necessitating an additional mixing operation. The pearls are normally added after the binder has been uniformly distributed throughout the batch. Again, this is to minimize the work energy applied to the pearls. Some pearl coatings can handle the additional oils normally associated with the binder. In those cases, the pearls may be added before the binder. The lower energy of the "cutters," Table 13.6, compared to the hammer mill, can be used to disperse the binder with "minimal" effect on the pearls. The pearl may be added into the bulk in the same device used to perform the preliminary coarse mixing, providing the device has been cleaned.

It may sometimes be necessary to pass the bulk finally through a sieve or coarse screen to break up agglomerates of pearl and to ensure its even distribution. Some formulations use pearls that are processed through the hammer mill to develop a particular feel. Less expensive materials should always be evaluated, if this is required for a successful product, rather than purchase specialty-sized particles designed to impart appearance effects that are then resized to meet physical and not visual aesthetics. A minimum of energy should be applied to pearls to maximize their benefit to the product while minimizing the cost of the product.

Treated pigments and pearls may allow additional flexibility to the formulation since less processing should be required to attain particular aesthetics. As an example, a lower binder level may be used in a high-pearl formula (making for easier processing with less milling) because the treated/coated particles accept the wet binder easier with fewer spots and streaks.

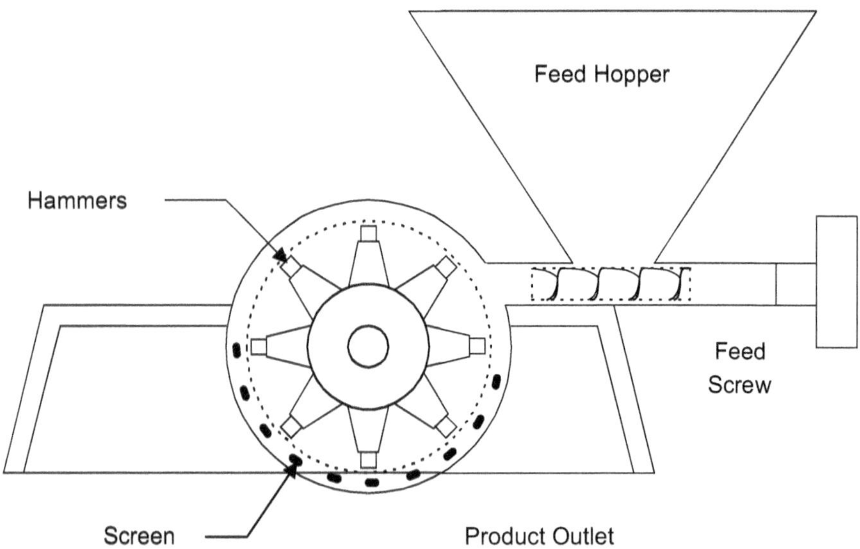

Figure 13.32: Hammer Mill

b. Shearing Equipment

The hammer mill was designed as a comminution, particle-size reduction machine. The standard design consists of a fast-rotating shaft fitted with freely swinging hammers mounted in a cage that is equipped with a breaker plate against which the feed is disintegrated, chiefly by impact from the hammers. The very high speed at which the hammers move (60–80 m s^{-1}) increases the chance of a hammer making contact with each particle and with particles making contact with particles. The dwell-time of particles within the chamber is controlled by the placement of different-size screens over the exit. Alternate designs exist that have different hammer designs or no swinging hammers with the rotor being a single unit. The alternate designs offer some cleaning benefits because the disassembly is easier and simpler.

Hammer mills are very efficient in the comminuting of brittle particles in the range of 1500–50 micron, but below this size their efficiency (the probability of direct impact) falls off rapidly. This is fortunate, since it means that small-particle-size cosmetic talcs and micas (not pearls or pearl extensions) can be passed through without being substantially altered. At the same time, however, the very high rotational speed of the hammers and the airflow within the chamber ensure that there are enough weak secondary impacts (particle-wall and particle-particle) to break the much weaker pigment agglomerates—which may be up to 500 micron in diameter. The primary particle size for most pigments is 0.1 micron in diameter. The mill is primarily a de-agglomeration device. The disintegrated agglomerate fractions then stabilize by becoming coated onto larger talc or mica particles and should not be further changed by subsequent passes through the mill equipped with the same screen. The tip-speed of the mill should be controlled to ensure that its energy level is higher than any other energy level developed during subsequent processing. For example, if a batch of powder is initially milled through a coarse screen for color development and then milled through a fine screen for improved binder dispersion (at the same tip speed), the shade of the product will change. This is because the pre-milled colors will see a higher level of energy once the binder is added and the batch is milled. The addition of binders may aid in the development of color; however, the quantity of energy and type of equipment used will determine the possible particle-size distribution that will be produced.

Nevertheless the hammer mill, in its role as an extender of pigments onto talc or other substrates, has certain disadvantages. For example, most of the extremely high energy it makes available is wasted and is largely dissipated in heating the powder. From the viewpoint of energy consumption, a hammer mill is very inefficient. The feed-rate and therefore the processing time for all but the smallest batch sizes of powder is very slow. The screen size is adjustable, but one does not set the screen at the size particle that is needed. The finest screen is normally 0.010-inch (0.254 mm) wide slits approximately 0.5 inches (12.7 mm) long in a herringbone pattern.

An attempt to speed up the process by the substitution of exit screens of larger diameter opening reduces the residence time in the mill. This often results in inadequate extension, necessitating a second, third, or fourth pass through the mill. On the other hand, increasing the residence time of powder within the grinding chamber by decreasing this opening size can cause the screen to become blocked with compacted and bridged powder, resulting in overheating and damage to both the machine and product. The design of the hammer mill allows a high volume of air to pass through it during the milling operation. This airflow can assist in minimizing a temperature rise during processing, but it cannot eliminate it. The airflow will also cause a fraction, usually less than 2% of what is being milled to be lost as fines (small particles that are easily carried through the air-handling system). If the process is not properly adjusted, the losses can be as high as 30%. If this high level of milling is required for the process, an alternate high-shear device should be examined, like the jet-mill, turbine mill, or classifier mill.

Perhaps the biggest disadvantage of all is that the hammer mill is a noisy, continuous processing device being used for batch processing. Since it is a continuous process device, it must be fed with a powder mixture that has already been effectively mixed, otherwise the color of the product exiting the mill will change as each section of unmixed bulk passes through. This preliminary mixing must be efficient, particularly if there is minimal mixing during the subsequent processing. It is not necessary for any extension to be achieved at this stage. The formulator will normally include an excess of the substrate material in this sequence to ensure a complete extension of the pigments. Subsequent blending will then be used to produce a uniform finished product.

The hammer mill has a design flaw that must be remembered. Some powder can drop vertically through the unit without being affected by the rotating hammers. It is typical, when milling pigments, to pass the batch through the hammer mill at least two times to increase the probability that all particles are hit and extended at least once. Alternate milling designs may have the same design problem or exit from a side or top panel to minimize this concern.

c. Alternatives to the Hammer Mill

The drawbacks to the hammer mill, as used for powder extension, have led to a search for other machines that can fulfill this function more satisfactorily. The ideal equipment would probably have the following properties:

- It would be capable of breaking up weak particles in the size range 0.5–50 μm without damaging talc or mica particles of similar diameter.
- It would be a low-energy device, consuming little power itself without heating the powder mixture excessively.
- It would be both a batch- and continuous-processing device capable of mixing and extending in one operation.
- It would be rapid: processing times of less than 10 minutes for 100 kilograms.
- It would not cause aeration of the powder (since this causes problems in later processing).

- Its efficiency would not vary with the cohesiveness of the powder—it would not be affected by poor flow characteristics of the raw materials.
- It would be quiet, clean in operation, and easy to clean.

Other comminution devices have been shown to produce extension. Pin mills (inefficient when compared to a hammer mill) and fluid energy or jet mills (too efficient at particle-size reduction when compared to a hammer mill) are two examples. No alternative seems to work as efficiently as the hammer mill at spreading the pigment onto the talc or mica.

In recent years, however, the development of high-speed powder mixers, which are also capable of producing some degree of extension, has brought the industry closer to the ideal. Two types in particular are worth mentioning. The first of these is best described as the horizontal vortex mixer. As an alternate high-speed mixer, it is often referred to as a plough-shear device, because of the unusual shape of the mixing paddles, which rotate on an axial shaft in a cylindrical-like horizontal mixing chamber (similar to a ribbon blender). These paddles cause the powder from all parts of the chamber to be thrown about in such a way that it all passes rapidly through a zone occupied by a series of rapidly revolving blades off a separate shaft referred to as a "chopper." The chopper is largely responsible for the powder extension and may be switched on or off independently of the main axial drive.

The second type is a high-speed modified bowl granulator. It has a propeller- or anchor-shaped blade of "good aerodynamic" design that rotates very rapidly in the dished base of the mixing bowl. This design mixer has a separate "chopper" shaft to increase the available energy to extend the pigments. Mixing and dispersion occur at the point of collision of the powder particles (in the upper part of the mixing bowl) by particle-particle and chopper-particle collisions. The flow pattern in modified bowl granulation vessels must be properly scaled from the laboratory through the pilot plant and into production. Specific batch sizes, with less than 20% powder loading, are required to maintain the proper flow characteristics. The tip speeds are usually matched for all of the process sizes being utilized. This will help to control the time factors in scale-up. Often, special designs are required to ensure scale-up including upgraded motor controls and blade speed operating ranges.

Both types of mixer have been used as partial or complete replacements for the traditional blender-hammer mill combination. Variations of these mixers have also been used in the solids-liquids processing area.

d. Batch Color Correction

It is not unusual for the bulk powder product, even though it has been correctly processed, to require color correction in order to obtain a satisfactory match to the standard. Since any addition of pigment or talc may need to be extended, a passage through the mill is necessary. A common procedure is as follows: After the preliminary process has been completed, a small quantity of the bulk (usually 2–5 kilograms), which is assumed to be representative of the whole, is passed through the mill with a coarse screen (≥ 0.125"). (This is to simulate the final milling step in a typical powder process.) This is examined in the laboratory, and if necessary, a pigment addition specified. This correction is added to the small quantity of the bulk product, mixed in roughly by hand, and the small quantity is re-milled through a fine screen (between 0.010" and 0.035"), twice. The screen size matches the one used during the original process. The twice-milled sample is returned to the remainder of the batch and remixed in the original mixer. A further sample is then removed and the process is repeated until a match is obtained. This method works well as long as the formula can handle the additional pigment without affecting the "feel" or other specifications (testing for international markets or for drug products requires an alternate adjusting method). The finished formula rarely matches the 100% formula originally developed by the Chemist.

There are a number of minor variations to this procedure, which are adapted to suit individual companies; the most important of these is the use of pigments previously extended on talc or mica and stored as such. This has the merit of speeding up the correction process by only requiring the extension to be blended into the batch without the fine screen milling to eliminate particle specks or streaks.

Full formula extenders are used throughout the industry to ensure that adjusted batches continue to match the 100% formula. However, this requires the production area to produce at least five additional batches, depending upon the pigments used in the formula—typically white, red, yellow, black, and colorless. The colorless extender is to "base out" the batch if the shade is too intense. This method is particularly useful if the extenders can also be blended together to make small batches of some shades, which provides some additional flexibility to production. The equipment necessary to make a full batch may be more elaborate than the equipment necessary to blend extenders (typically no high-shear device is required to produce the finished blend).

Another adjustment protocol uses adjusting base(s). This is a full formula extender without the pigment (or pearls). The pigment (and pearl) is added and usually milled into this base, keeping the ratios of the formula constant. This now-full formula extender is added to the batch for adjustment. Now, only one additional batch is required for production to make and store. The use of an adjusting base will be determined by the formula. If the formula without pigment is too wet, the adjusting base will not store well (see Bulk Powder Storage). Separate adjusting bases may also be needed for pearl and nonpearl shades. The first adjusting method described is the simplest, but it may produce the most batch-to-batch variations in final formulas.

When pearl agents are part of the formulation, unless an unpearlized standard is provided, the pearl must be added in the correct proportion to the laboratory sample before color can be assessed. Pearl is normally added to the bulk in the last stage of the manufacturing procedure. Adjusting the shade of a product is often very difficult due to the lighting effects of the pearl. It is important to train the operator on physical and visual examination of the product. The use of light boxes, as a controlled lighting source, is also important. However, it is critical that a standard method of evaluation be maintained from the development stage through the Quality Assurance evaluation of finished goods.

e. Powder Grinds for Creams and Lotions Batches—Dry Mix

If milling of the pigments in a liquid media is not available due to the formula parameters, a dry mix may be needed by Production to shade a cream or lotion batch. The logistics of this type of process requires multiple awkward controls without gaining improved shade control of the finished mass. The procedure is outlined as follows:

1. A batch of the cream or lotion is made without the pigment. This batch must be acceptable from all stability parameters, as it will be used to adjust the shade of the pigment blend.
2. A pigment batch is made. This includes mixing and milling of the pigments and filler powders until a drawdown shows no color specks or streaks.
3. A quantity of the pigment-free bulk is blended with the pigment grind. The same mixing as in production should be scaled for this operation (usually about one liter, similar to the formulation laboratory).
4. The finished laboratory batch is compared to the standard.
5. The appropriate shade adjustment is made on the pigment blend, including milling.
6. Steps 3 through 5 are repeated until the pigment batch produces a finished batch that matches standard.

The powder grind is then used in the actual production of the finished product. Since the powder was pre-matched, no shade adjustment should be required. If these operations—pigment processing and finished cream or lotion production—are performed at different locations, a great deal of finger pointing may ensue if a batch is made without matching the standard. Sometimes a specially colored, full-size production batch will need to be made and blended with the batch that does not match standard to minimize color variations. The use of a dry-mix process is to be discouraged during all phases of the development and production of the finished product.

f. Loose Powders

Loose powder production uses similar equipment and follows a similar process to that of pressed powders. The blending operation is relatively simple with little high-shear energy needed—except for some preservatives, a little color, and for the addition of oil or fragrance. The requirements for chemical uniformity are lower (from a specifications standpoint) for a loose powder than for a pressed powder. The loose powder is usually examined as a gross or large-quantity powder. The pressed powder (cake or tablet) is usually examined based upon the actives or the pickup from a brush or sponge.

Particle-size distribution and the associated handling concerns are usually more critical with a loose powder than with a pressed powder. Inhalation concerns will often require the formula and process to be very specific and therefore limit the Chemist on flexibility of formula. Oils and waxes may be added to the formula to intentionally agglomerate the finer particles due to limited availability of raw materials with the preferred (safer) particle-size distribution. This addition may be performed as a side phase and added to the main batch as a previously processed ingredient.

The packages for loose powders are larger than those of pressed powders. Therefore, larger batch sizes are normally produced for loose powders. Loose powders may contain a small pigment phase that requires milling, but most do not. Even high levels of fragrance usually do not require a great deal of milling since if the mass is too wet, it will agglomerate and no longer be loose. Without the need for higher energy during processing, less efficient mixing systems can be used by production. The batching times for these large, loose powder batches may be longer than for a similar formula pressed powder. The oldest, slowest machines are usually saved by production for loose powder work. Most loose powders are fragranced, while most pressed powders are not. Removing fragrance from equipment can be very challenging and difficult. Large batch sizes and simplified quality testing ensure that a small quantity of residual fragrance has a minimal effect on the next batch to be processed.

g. Filling Loose Powders

Loose powder filling machine or auger fillers are used to fill non–free-flowing powder into containers. This type of equipment is relatively low maintenance and gives high-accuracy filling. The machine works both on auto or manual configuration. It consists of a hopper equipped with sweep blade connecting to an auger. As the blades turn, the powder moves inside the hopper and the auger displaces the product through the funnel into the container held under the dispensing nozzle. The electronic sensor provides the precise filling cycle through an enclosed pulley unit, brake, and clutch that is fixed on auger shaft. Once the sensor sends signals, the powder filler machine will fill-in the automated quantity of powder product into the container through the auger. The two designs either start and stop through a timed cycle or based upon a particular number of revolutions of the auger screw. Cosmetics loose powder containers are usually plastic jars.

An alternate filling system pulls a vacuum on the filling container. The level of vacuum is controlled to "pull" the powder into the container to meet the proper weight. The powder must be free-flowing for this type of filler. If the vacuum seal is not perfect, the packages will get dusty from overfill.

Filling is dependent upon the flow characteristics of the powder. Rotary volumetric fillers are used to fill powders at high production rates. These systems are designed to enable the powder to freely flow into moving chambers that control the weight and/or volume of powder to be filled. The chambers are designed to completely release the pre-set quantity of product into the package (usually boxes or bags) just prior to sealing the package. Automatic dishwashing detergents, powdered bath products, and cereals are packaged this way. Due to variations in bulk density that may be enhanced through shipping, these packages are completely opaque and are typically labeled "Note that settling may occur during shipping and storage." The volumetric filling system design can tightly control fill variation of the package assuming the variation of powder to be minimal.

h. Filling Pressed Powders

There are several different types of press powder machines available. Most machines are equipped with powder feed system that use a linear-vibratory feed or free-flowing feed to supply the pans with loose powder to be pressed. Hand distribution of powders into the cavities with pans is a key variable to be continually examined by the Chemist and Quality Assurance. Although hand "raking" of powder can be very efficient, slight variations in loading into a pan can give very different aesthetics. The Chemist will often weigh powder for individual pans being pressed. The production variations need to be understood when providing samples for evaluation. All the presses can produce acceptable tablets within the pressure range of 100 to 1000 psig (6 to 70 bar). It is important to remember that the pressure across a single pan is not the same pressure across several pans unless the total surface area remains constant. Different pressing systems are as follows:

- **Top-down press:** This is an automated powder press machine that is normally used for large-quantity runs. It is used for pressing face powder, eye shadow, or blush into pans. It is designed in a manner that the single or multiple punch press driven by hydraulic or electric piston from top moves down to stationary module where pan is located. Pressing cloth is normally fed from a roll.
- **Bottom-up press:** The mold moves up and is driven by piston into single or multiple stationary punches. This style of pressing helps the powder to deaerate better than the top-down method. Deaeration depends on the ribbon cloth and the gradual pressure applied until the target pressure is

achieved. Pressing cloth is normally placed manually in single sheets. This press machine is used for face powder or eye shadow.

- **Manual press:** This is a single-press machine that is used for small runs. It is also used for blush and eye shadow that are pressed into unusually shaped pans. This single-pan application operates with manual pump via hydraulic piston to press the powder pan. To regulate the amount of pressure applied on the powder, a pressure gauge installed on the press reads the pressure of the top punch when pressing on the mold pan area. The pumping should stop when the desired pressure is achieved.

The design of the manual press is such that usually the punch is driven downward to the stationary mold with loose powder in the pan. However, in a laboratory unit, the bottom plate moves up with the loose powder in a pan and the punch is stationary.

All of the different systems used to produce pressed powders have certain components in common. The powder must be presented to the filler. The appropriate cavity is filled and the cavity is placed under pressure. The pressed unit is collected, tested, and placed in a package for shipping.

In presenting the powder to the filler, it must be uniformly presented to each pan. This may require that a "fluffing" be performed just prior to filling. This fluffing may be as simple as rolling the drums of powder before use to evenly aerate the mass. It may be as formal as a container with a mixing blade designed to aerate the powder as it travels to the filler. It may be an air conveyor system that aerates the powder as it is moved. Aeration is not a preferred action, since the air must be pressed out of the powder in the next step. However, the change in density after storage may be necessary to achieve uniform production at the press over multiple shifts.

Variations in tablet press quality may be due to flexing of the structure, cycle rate, internal pressure measurement, pan variability, and fill variability. Formulation will affect very few of these variables. However, it is important for the formulator to understand the variability of the press during formulation. If the pressing pressure range for an acceptable tablet is too small, due to the acceptance of other characteristics (payoff, coverage/sheerness, packing density/durometer, size and shape of pan, type of applicator, etc.) good production runs will not be the norm. A small variation in the pressing pressure should not produce a significant change in the aesthetics. The formula may not need to be adjusted, but an acceptable pressure range may be required.

Pharmaceutical tablet and soap pressing are separate specialty presses. Pharmaceutical tablet presses are designed for near continuous operation and can be used to generate over 10,000 psig (667 bar). They can produce over 10,000 tablets a minute using dual-station operation, depending upon the tablet size. Since these are normally used in the pharmaceutical industry only, the tablet is not pressed into a pan. Similar controls are needed to those of the pressed eye shadow, but the flow characteristics are much more critical. The small volumes must be filled easily and consistently to provide the correct level of drug/active to each tablet. Improper settings will very quickly force thousands of dollars worth of materials to be rejected.

Sometimes, the powders will be partially agglomerated to better control their flow through the production system. Pressing times are still an issue, so production machines are often rotary with the rotating table being very large to provide sufficient pressing/dwell time for each tablet. Soap pressing may be performed at very low pressures, which are both formula and package dependent. The slurry of bar soap is injected (sometimes using an extruder) into a mold, minimizing uncontrolled air while the bar shape is formed. The soap bars are then dried and packaged. Molds are typically brass or sometimes stainless steel. There are periodic uses in cosmetics, like bath and toilet bowl additives, that have smaller production requirements. The key part for both of these presses is the control of the process from raw materials through the exit of the press. Since production is continuous, any delay in testing or uncontrolled operation can ruin huge quantities of finished goods.

Parameters used to control pressed powder products:

- Target pressure: This element plays a balancing act in keeping the powders together in a tablet form in order to pass and meet the general QA tests standards, such as drop test, payoff, and texture.
- Press/dwell time: The press time is critical to form a tablet and deaerate the powder to be pressed, and it normally ranges between half a second to two seconds in order to complete the pressing cycle. The dwell time is the hold at the maximum pressure to ensure the pressed tablet does not bounce back after compression. An extended dwell time can sometimes produce a different product feel. This does not usually affect the product, but it is an operation that may be a variable for the press. Any increase in dwell time is a decrease in production capacity.
- **Mixer/augur speed:** The augur positioned inside the holding tank helps to move the powder towards the dispensing nozzle. The longer the rotation time, the more consistent powder is dispensed, but the more the powder may have pre-compacted producing flow issues.
- **Type of pressing ribbon:** The type of ribbon used is driven by aesthetic and press deaeration. The pattern and weave of the ribbon cloth is selected based on several reasons such as type of powder, aesthetic appearance, and desired final quality. The weave of the cloth (threads per inch [or millimeter] and the size [diameter] of the threads) is used to produce a consistent

texture across the finished pan. The tighter-weave ribbon provides better aesthetic with finer finish but at the same time traps air inside the pressed tablet, which may cause a spongy look and breakage. The more moderate weave or less coarse ribbon cloth helps the powder to deaerate during press. It also provides better payoff and texture; however, the aesthetic may not be as pleasing since it leaves a larger print pattern on the pressed tablet. If the mass contains too much air for the cloth to vent, the pressed piece may immediately crumble once the pressure is removed or it may bow as the air bubbles in the powder are released from being under pressure. If the pressing cloth is too fine for the air to release, a second press may be necessary. In normal operation, the pressing cloth is changed and the press is operated a second time. Some automated machines can perform these two presses at different pressures to best control the density of the powder throughout the pan—start low, finish high. This double operation will cut production capacity by approximately 40%.

- **Press number:** Some products require multiple pressing to achieve the desired characteristics. Usually the first press is done at a lower pressure to dissipate the air and the second press applied at a higher force or target pressure to achieve the final formed tablet. (Some tests have been done by the equipment vendors to validate the finished pressure from multiple presses. The results indicate no change in pressure value, but possibly less aeration in the finished press.)
- The design of the mold and die will determine the net pressure available for each pan, and therefore the capacity limitations. Different pan materials hold and dispel static charge differently. Most pans are steel or aluminum (if water is involved in the formula or the end use). Some pans are plastic. The handling characteristics are very different. Pan shape and depth will affect the flow of the powder prior to and during the pressing operation. Sharp corners make for easy breakage. Round pans handle high pressures more evenly across the entire surface.

i. Powder Scale-Up—Batch

Scale-up of powders is dependent upon many processing parameters. These include the following, which must be measured and controlled from the laboratory bench, through the pilot plant, and throughout production.

- the batch loading by volume and/or by weight [to be maintained]—which affects the flow patterns in the compounding vessel
- the shear being imparted on the powders and powder dispersions (typically measured as tip speed) [to be maintained]—which affect the color

and color development of the raw materials

- the process time [to be scaled or maintained]—which affects the overall production capacity
- the batching temperatures [to be maintained]—improper processing can produce temperature elevations of over 40°C from the normal batching temperature
- the batching procedure [to be scaled or maintained]—due to the use of high-shear, detailed procedures will maintain the quantity of shear consistently through all production
- the sequencing of the phases [to be maintained]—changes in sequence will affect the color or intensity and consumer characteristics ("feel") of the finished product
- the raw materials [to be maintained or at least controlled]—examples: (1) variations in dye strengths, in different lots of pigments, will change the finished shades and require color adjustments; (2) changes in particle-size distributions will change the look of larger-particle pearls; (3) changes in the source may shift the color range from red with yellow to red with blue

Batch loading, the quantity of powder to be produced in a given vessel configuration, is a particular problem for all new formulas. If a new shade is being made of an existing product, a history through production has already been developed. A new product may be less dense, more cohesive, more brittle, contain a higher pigment load, a higher binder level, a higher pearl level, or be more temperature sensitive and harder to press than a formula already in production. All of these variables can affect the batch loading. If the loading is too high, the process will usually create a higher intermediate temperature during processing. The spraying characteristics (spray pattern and particle-size distribution) of the binder will also be affected if a constant addition time is to be maintained; the flow rate will be changing as the process scales-up. If the batch is being milled *in situ*, using a bowl granulator for instance, the loading will significantly affect the color development. Unfortunately, multiple laboratory, pilot, and production batches may be required to determine and fine-tune the proper loading.

Process time has some additional flexibility with powders that is not usually available in liquid systems. Since heating and cooling are not usually taking place during the mixing or shearing operation, the actual time necessary for a step to take place is less critical. However, the steps should be performed in a very consistent manner with times that can be duplicated. If the scale-up time from the laboratory to the pilot plant for one product is one to ten, it should be maintained for all similar products that use the same equipment system. If it is not, some process variable is not being controlled and could become a major problem for production.

The development of accurate and detailed procedures is key to proper color development and shade matching of products. The protocols used to evaluate finished bulk, finished/packaged products, and, where necessary, intermediate sequences must be as controlled as is the equipment being used. Evaluation of esthetics can be difficult to translate to an intermediate process test. Standard measurements of rotational speed, temperature, and time may be all that is available. These may be sufficient. In addition, motor current draw, on a high- or low-shear drive, may be used to indicate that a spray addition was uneven or that a batching scale is out of calibration. Both of these problems would make for batches that would be a challenge to shade match as well as an increased opportunity to produce rejected product. New pieces of equipment used to measure powder flow characteristics have recently been introduced to the pharmaceutical and cosmetics markets. These instruments can provide some numerical indicators on flow and shear during development and production of powder phases and batches.

Production may schedule work as a series of batches. An example for loose powders may be based upon fragrance intensities (light level or scent to heavy). They may schedule a series of pressed powders batches based upon color intensities (white to yellow to red to black/dark). These scheduling groups can help Production to minimize the effects of a poorly cleaned system or an elaborate cleaning procedure. Some of the newer equipment designs allow Clean-In-Place (CIP) operation. (CIP is an automated system for cleaning equipment following an exact protocol the same way every time. It should only be used when a system is designed and tested to ensure that proper controls make the system clean every time. New products should always be "validated.") Most of the older equipment, notably the ribbon blender, cannot be CIPed due to the design limitations of its sealing systems, which may leak and may not be very water-friendly. Cleaning of a ribbon blender can be a slow, tedious process and is rarely 100% effective.

Production schedules can minimize the effects of this problem. To meet other regulatory requirements, equipment (batching vessels and sometimes mills, weighing areas, and compounding areas) is often designated for organic pigments only or inorganic pigments only.

Powder systems, with their inherently low water level (activity) are rarely a microbiological problem. However, the use of preservatives is included in most formulas due to the package design and the methods of use by the consumer. Even if the equipment has not been completely cleaned before the next batch, it must be sanitized. This may produce "clean" dirt, but the finished product will not be a site for potential microbial growth while the consumer uses the product. The newer systems that allow CIP usually also allow SIP (Sanitization-In-Place). The preferred method is to use steam. The residual heat will dry the vessel. Chemicals may also be used for sanitization, but these could leave a residual and affect the next product.

13.1.7.1 WET CONTINUOUS PROCESS

The objective of building a continuous process, as compared to the batch processes discussed earlier, for an emulsion, liquid/liquid, or liquid/solid cosmetic product is generally the need for high-volume production. It may also be desired for just-in-time manufacture or to make a special product where intense energy is required to form a viscous product such as a hair-styling gel. Examples of the most common cosmetic products made via this method include hydro-alcoholics, creams, lotions, shampoos, hair conditioners, hair dye developers, and hair-styling gels. Color cosmetics, such as liquid or cream makeup, may also be possible provided color correction is not required.

Formula composition is maintained using stoichiometric calculations usually by means of a series of piston pumps, connected by a common shaft with a variable-speed motor/drive. Piston pumps are generally used to allow for higher pressures with accurate delivery. Each phase in the formula requires a separate pump to control its composition in the total formula. Each pump is calibrated for weight delivery by adjusting its stroke length at a constant motor/drive speed. This will lock that ingredient or phase into the proper formulation. Production rate is then increased or decreased by speeding up or slowing down the drive motor. Pumps employed may be of several designs depending upon the application. Sanitary pulsation dampeners may be employed downstream to smooth out flow, but oftentimes are not necessary. Other components of the process may include some or all of the following items:

- a static mixer for pre-mixing some or all of the formulation constituents
- a dynamic mixer to provide additional mixing energy to set the emulsion or dispersion
- a scraped-wall, plate-and-frame, or tubular heat exchanger to cool the product if required

The final components in the system prior to storage or filling are usually pH or conductivity and viscosity in-line measuring. This equipment is used to monitor quality. They will usually control adjusted pump delivery to maintain the finished product specifications or sound an alarm to shut the system down. The complete process may be freestanding and require considerable space, or mounted on portable skids and rolled up to a production filling line for just-in-time manufacture depending on the complexity of the design, size, and application.

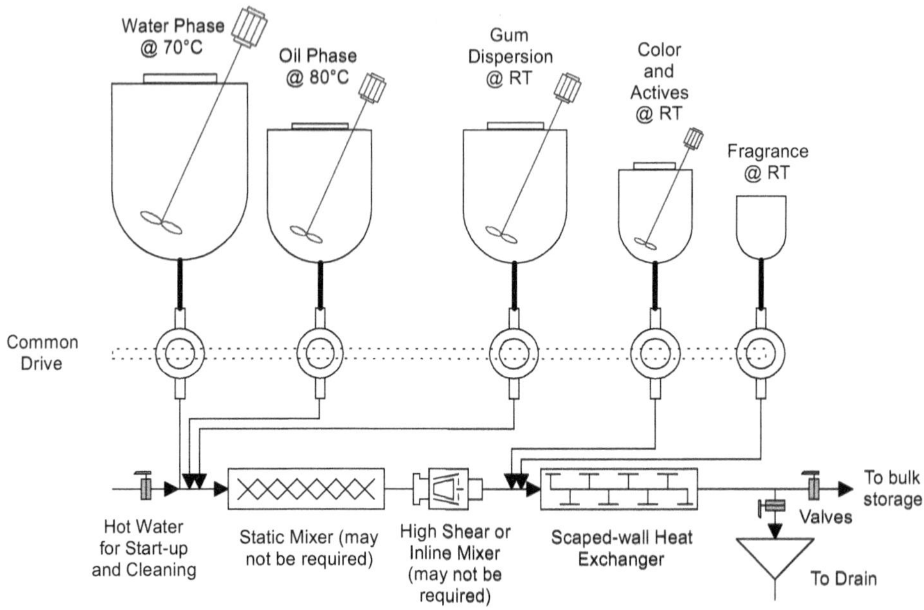

Figure 13.33: Simple Continuous Process Liquids System

a. Emulsion Products Requiring Cooling

Experience has shown that for lotions, creams, etc., it is usually possible to form a crude emulsion by metering the oil and water phases and gum phase first into a static mixer, Figure 13.33. The crude emulsion is then finished either in a dynamic in-line mixer and/or a scraped-wall heat exchanger where other temperature sensitive colors, fragrances, and actives are injected just before the heat exchanger inlet. This minimizes their exposure to heat to just a few seconds during the rapid cooling process within the heat exchanger. Injected ingredients should be added into the centerline of the pipe at a velocity equal to the mass velocity of the formula passing that point. This will minimize concentration pockets in the stream. The advantage of the scraped-wall heat exchanger is that it can be used as a final mixing element by controlling its internal shaft speed (mutator) during very rapid cooling to set product rheology prior to storage and/or filling. Cooling capacity and rate is very high in these units, being four to five times more efficient and substantially more rapid than cooling in a CSTR. Some products, however, cannot tolerate the turbulence and/or cooling rate produced in these units. Plate-and-frame or tubular heat exchangers may be employed where cooling rate is less critical and can be slower. Product viscosities are usually low, so films do not build up in the heat exchanger and limit temperature control. These can also be used when mixing energy during cooling is detrimental to product rheology.

There are two things to keep in mind when one needs to make an existing batch-made product on a continuous flow process.

(1) The continuous-made emulsion will have a smaller mean average particle size and a much narrower particle-size distribution compared to the batch-made product. This may change product rheology and affect such things as rub-in break and feel on the skin. This occurs because every particle of the continuously made product is exposed to much more uniform mixing energy than is possible in batch-made product. Experience has shown, however, that through careful tuning of the continuous process, the rheological properties can be brought close enough to those made by batch process so that the consumer cannot detect a significant difference.

(2) One should be aware that continuous-made product, particularly lotions, may have a much lower initial viscosity, perhaps as low as 20% of that compared to initial batch-made product. This is due once again to the intense mixing energy imparted in either the in-line mixer and/or the scraped-wall heat exchanger. However, the rate of viscosity build may be much faster achieving the same value as the initial batch viscosity within the first two or three hours. This may require that the product be stored for several hours prior to filling to prevent filling issues like a premature shutoff of the filling nozzles. This would produce uneven fills due to rapid viscosity changes during filling. Normally, the product equilibrium viscosity will reach the same value as batch-made product within a few days, if total and finishing work energy in the heat exchanger (mutator shaft speed and velocity of product) have been respected.

b. Emulsion Hair Conditioners

Emulsion hair conditioners may require much more sensitive temperature control during the process prior to filling or storage than that of most other products. A typical arrangement for this type of product would require the following in sequence:

- heated oil phase
- heated water phase
- metering pumps for the above
- static mixer
- plate-and-frame heat exchanger—a simple design that is easy to maintain with excess area to control the exit temperature of the crude emulsion to within ± 0.5°C of a predetermined intermediate temperature (temperature is chosen based upon DSC curves and set point of oil-phase ingredients)
- dynamic mixer (typically rotor/stator)—used to set the product rheology at that temperature

- another plate-and-frame heat exchanger—to cool the product prior to storage or filling
- backpressure valve—to control the residence time in the dynamic mixer
- in-line pH and viscosity instrumentation and mix systems—used to monitor product quality, adjust phases, or note alarm conditions and shut the system down

It should be noted that the use of a scraped-wall heat exchanger would not work in this application due to destruction of the product viscosity at lower temperatures. Experimental work is required to determine the correct temperature of feed to the dynamic mixer combined with the correct rotor/stator configuration, speed, backpressure, and product flow rate, to obtain the desired results prior to scale-up.

c. Hair Gels

Hair gels are generally processed cold. They consist of a water phase containing polymers and styling agents, and a solvent phase containing neutralizer, colorants, and other desired ingredients. These phases are generally metered together at room temperature into a static mixer to form a crude gel followed by a dynamic mixer to complete the gel structure. The finished gel then passes through in-line pH and viscosity instrumentation prior to filling or storage. Instrumentation can be provided to adjust the neutralizer phase pump based on pH feedback and/or viscosity. Experimental work is required to develop process parameters such as the number of static mixing elements required, flow rate, dynamic mixing speed, backpressure required for different production rates, and phase tolerances required, ensuring control of the formulation.

d. Scale-Up of Continuous Systems

A pilot system producing between 0.5 and 5 kilograms per minute of product containing all of the main components envisioned for the full-scale production system is recommended to work out the process. This size system lends itself well to the use of small commercial equipment. It can also demonstrate product characteristics and stability, determine operating parameters, and develop data for control of the process and the sizing of full-scale production equipment. In addition, it makes pilot runs of 30 minutes to two or more hours reasonable to handle to examine formula and/or process changes.

The pilot system should be designed with maximum flexibility built into each component of the process. This will allow collection of scale-up data over the entire operating range. The system would include such things as variable-speed drives on phase pumps, dynamic mixers, and scraped-wall heat exchangers.

Sufficient instrumentation should also be provided to ensure accurate recording of temperature, pressures, and speeds of dynamic equipment during experimental runs so that material and energy balances can be calculated for each component. The following scale-up rules to keep in mind:

- pipelines should be sized for equal velocities and pressure drop
- static mixers should be the same style and contain the same number of elements
- dynamic in-line mixers should have the same rotor/stator design, number of stages, variable-speed drives, and rotor tip speeds where possible
- scraped-wall, plate-and-frame, or tubular heat exchangers should be connected for overall countercurrent heat transfer for maximum efficiency and sized to match developmental parameters—equal velocity throughput, residence time, mutator shaft tip speed where applicable, and overall heat transfer coefficient

The data, when supplied to the engineering department and the equipment manufacturer, will aid substantially in getting the proper full-scale equipment specified and in place. The production equipment typically will not have the same flexibility as the pilot system. Changes to the production system can usually be justified when the next product is developed. By controlling the flexibility/components of the production system, fewer errors occur during the life of the product, producing a more consistent product for the consumer.

e. Production Design Considerations

If heated or cooled phases are required in the process it is necessary to trace, insulate, and control the temperature of pipelines from the bottom of the heated phase tanks to and including the metering pumps and the return lines to the top of the phase tanks for weight calibration purposes. Tandem phase tanks may be required for water and oil phases, etc., since materials must be melted, dissolved, or chilled. One phase tank is thus "online" while the other is being prepared. The alternative to this is to size the vessels for a shift or more of production. In some cases it may also be necessary to control the temperature of phase lines on the pump discharge leading to the point where the initial emulsion or dispersion is formed in order to prevent "salting out" or solidification in lines. The need for this must be determined in the pilot plant.

If the product requires "aging" to ensure conformity to specifications, bulk storage of mass may be required. If so, capacity should be based upon the longest age time and testing that may be required (the storage tanks may not be upgradeable while the processing system can be).

Weight/mass calibration of each phase must be established at constant drive motor speed set at the actual flow conditions and line pressure that will occur during production. If the calibration is not performed at constant drive motor speed, the formula will not be correct once production starts. This requires installation of an adjustable valve in each recycle/calibration line to pressurize the pumps and recycle lines to ensure accurate calibration. Each recycle line should also have a check valve at the kettle return discharge point to keep the line full for weight accuracy. Suitable controls and instrumentation are required to allow flow to process or recycle for each phase independently, and to divert all phases to recycle or process simultaneously. These requirements are necessary to prime all process lines for calibration and production startup. An adjustable backpressure valve should be installed at the process end to keep pipelines full, control residence time, and optimize performance in the mixing and heat exchange equipment.

Once the stroke positions are set properly for each phase pump, calibration is complete. Startup is accomplished by first adjusting the drive motor to the selected speed and allowing the system to run in recycle mode under production line pressure conditions. Each phase process line is then primed to its injection point. Next, if heated phases and product cooling are required, the process portion of the system is made ready for product manufacture by passing hot water through the in-line mixers and heat exchangers (see Figure 39.35). This is necessary to bring the pipeline, mixers, and heat exchange equipment up to equilibrium conditions so that once the process is initiated a minimum of rework is created.

Production then begins by switching all pumps to process mode and simultaneously cutting off the hot water flow. Product exiting the heat exchangers is diverted to drain or reworked for a few seconds before allowing it to pass through the Quality Control in-line measuring equipment and into the storage or filling systems. This allows all the product temperature controls to reach equilibrium.

The system is shut down in reverse order as it was started up. Simultaneously the pumps are diverted into their recycle position; hot water is flushed through the pipeline, mixers, and heat exchangers and routed to the drain. This flushes the system in preparation for cleaning and sanitization for the next run. Supply and recycle lines from and to the heated phases and ingredient tanks are blown back to the tanks with air pressure, and are cleaned and sanitized as required.

13.1.7.2 DRY CONTINUOUS PROCESSING

Continuous production of powder products requires flexibility in the formula and large volumes for filling. Typical examples are powder water softeners, automatic dishwasher detergents, and bath products. In general, these products all share a few characteristics—they do not foam a great deal, they do not contain a large quantity of oils or other liquids, the powders are the active ingredients, and the raw materials all flow well, Figure 13.34.

The powder formula must be flexible to allow for a larger variation than with creams and lotions due to the different processing controls used in a continuous powder process. Typically, the raw materials are stored in bulk. Bulk storage expands the range of temperature and humidity the powders are subjected to compared with laboratory storage conditions. The ingredients for the formula are metered automatically or sub-phased as large batches to be used continuously. Therefore, only gross adjustments (color or fragrance level) can be made under controlled circumstances. Exact shades can rarely be reproduced. Even with modern process controls, the mixing systems will have normal variations. Without continuous in-line testing, finished product samples are grouped together for a general analysis. If the variations that resulted were unacceptable, recalls of finished goods would need to be made. This is a time-consuming and costly operation.

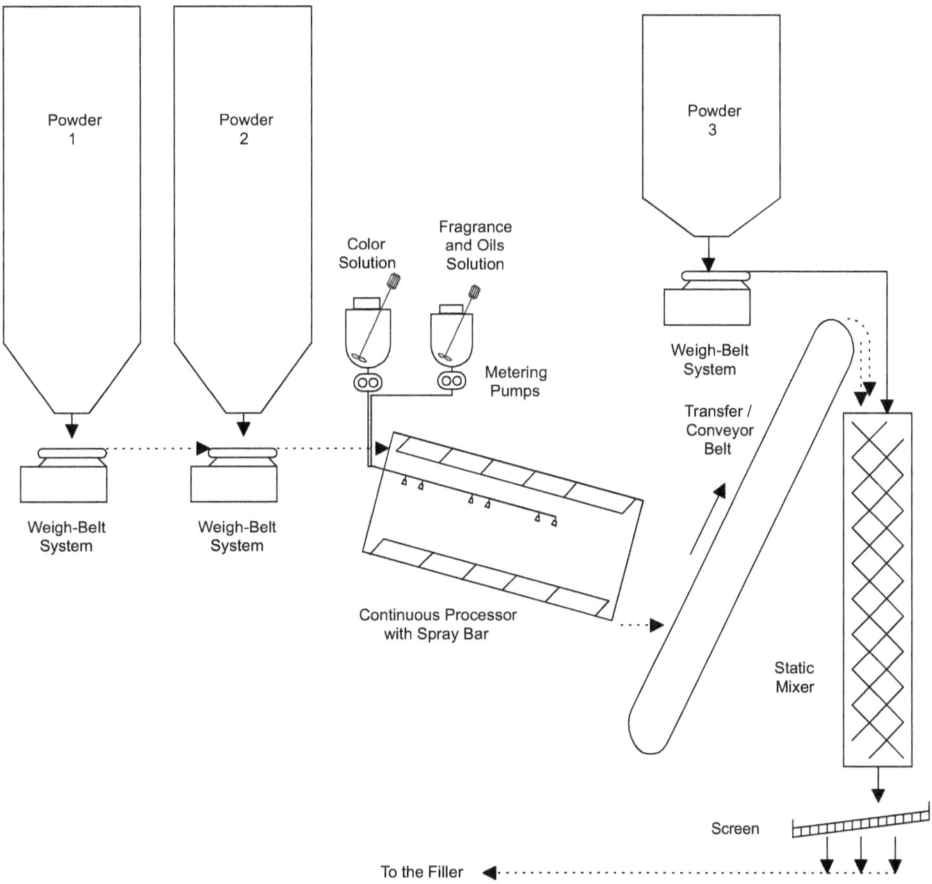

Figure 13.34: Simple Continuous Powder System

a. Bulk Powder Storage

The two factors that have an important effect on stored cosmetic powders are moisture and pressure. It is not always appreciated that a small increase in relative humidity can give rise to sufficient moisture in the stored powder to change the main mechanism of particle-particle bonding, which will increase the bond strength of agglomerates by a factor of 2 or more. Such an increase in cohesiveness can make the handling and flow problems already inherent in cosmetic powders perceptibly worse and can change the processing characteristics of (for instance) an eye shadow to the point where all the pressing machine settings may have to be altered to compensate.

In the same way, powder bulk that has been stored in vertical containers exhibits increasingly difficult flow characteristics as the container gradually empties. The lower layers, having been compressed by the weight of powder above them, become increasingly cohesive as the bottom is approached. If oils or moisture has been added to the powder, they may migrate towards the bottom of the container and produce a significant product change between the top and the bottom. For this reason, it is sometimes better to store powder blends in a large number of small, well-sealed containers than in loosely covered large bins. Each container should be mixed before removing any of its contents.

If the variability of the powders being stored is known, or at least controlled, the flow characteristics within a container can be adjusted through the design of the container. The most efficient design would have the first particle that was dropped in be the first particle that comes out (FIFO). Most simple silo designs do not function that well. Powders will settle towards the edges as fines while only a center core of material leaves the silo. This is termed funnel flow. Modifications to an existing silo are always cumbersome at best. Therefore, vibrators, or sometimes air jets are added to enhance the flow of material. Often, the operators use sledgehammers on the body of the silo or the outlet cone.

Design improvements have led towards an almost FIFO design called mass flow. Several variations have been designed, but they all require specific knowledge of the powders being stored, such as particle-size distribution, particle shape, density, angle of repose, etc. The angles of the sidewalls are designed to ensure that the particles cannot sit and accumulate. A change in the powder being handled may require a new silo, Figure 13.35.

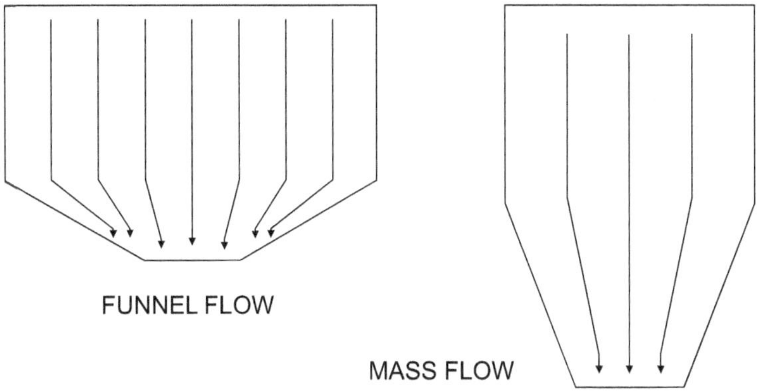

Figure 13.35: Hopper Flow

Mass flow versus funnel flow, as pictured above, shows the general physical difference of the two hopper/silo designs. The volumes and the outlet diameters are the same for the two hoppers shown in Figure 13.35. The funnel flow design will allow flow through a center core with finer particles gravitating towards the walls of the vessel. This will produce a change in particle-size distribution as the level in the hopper changes. It will also enable easier "bridging" of the outlet of agglomerated material. The mass flow hopper, by design, allows the lowest material to leave first while the top material leaves last. There is virtually no mixing or separation of the horizontal layers.

Often, the hopper supplier will design the slope of the sidewall to be sharper than a critical friction value for the particular material. As noted through the illustrations, the mass flow hopper is taller and narrower than the funnel flow design. If the hoppers are being installed to meet a particular volume requirement and there is a height limitation, a mass flow hopper may not be a true option. Alternate designs can be used to improve the flow characteristics of the silo; these designs modify the flow with internal changes, typically baffle plates. These alternate designs do not allow for complete cleaning without special attachments and will still have some particle-size distribution changes during use.

Industrial bulk containers (IBC), in an assortment of sizes, shapes, and materials of construction, are commonly used to store large volumes of powder. They can range in design from a large bag (sometimes with elaborate linings) to a skid-mounted silo. Since they hold less material than a "normal" silo, segregation due to particle size is less. These containers are normally filled at the supplier and emptied at the cosmetics manufacturing facility. Therefore, there is no concern that the first material received by the manufacturing facility will be the last out during use, as is the case in a poorly designed silo. It is assumed that the manufacturing facility will control the IBCs and use them FIFO. The key concern for the cosmetics and drug industries is contamination. Special bags have been designed to minimize sifting, which is the loss of powder at the seams of the bag. Sometimes, special one-piece liners are inserted into the bag to minimize sifting. It is assumed that if powder can come out, moisture and microbiological contamination can enter.

The cost of liners can be a problem. Single-use liners can be very expensive, but can be maintained microbiologically clean until use. Multiple-use liners may control sifting, but require cleaning and sanitization between uses. This may leave unwanted residuals in the bags, which can become incorporated into the next powder. The older, skid-mounted style containers are stainless steel and were originally designed to handle liquids (275 gallons in the same skid space as four 55-gallon drums). These containers do not work well with powders and often have cleaning and sanitization problems for liquid use. Newer designs can empty powders completely but the containers must be cleaned, sanitized, and dried before reuse. Microbiological concerns continue to exist for these containers.

Once the bulk container has been filled with powder, a transfer system is used to move the powders through the process. The typical conveyor systems fall into three main categories. The first design is pneumatic. An air blower is used to fluidize and then move the powders through special tubing. If the line sizes are not well matched to the flow rates, some segregation of particles may take place. If the powder must be kept dry, low-moisture air must be used to move the powder. This technique can be used to move large quantities of materials over very long distances with minimal product-to-product contact. Some particle-size breakdown takes place, which is often dependent upon the length of the run and the bends during the run. The second design is mechanical with product-to-product contact. A screw conveyor is a classic example of this technique. Another is a chain within a tube or housing. The screw is used to move the powder at a very controlled rate. By design, the distance between supply and deposit cannot be large. Since the movement of the screw or chain physically pushes or pulls the powder, degradation and compaction of the powder often take place. The third design is mechanical without product-to-product contact. Examples are bucket and belt conveyors. These conveyors move the powder in discrete increments with little detriment. Unfortunately, the atmospheric conditions must be controlled, particularly if moisture is a concern. This operation is usually open to the air, and microbial growth is always a finished-product concern.

All conveying systems have an inherent limitation when moving powders. Dust explosions can take place when dust levels reach a critical point within the conveyor operation or dust collector system. The explosions are actually deflagration (explosion with a propagation speed ranging between 0.1 and 100 meters per second, which generates pressure waves that are much faster than the flame front) not detonation (sudden burning without propagation). As with all burning conditions, oxygen and the combustible material must coexist along with an ignition source. The ignition source is often a static discharge or a worn or damaged component in the system. The combustible material is usually an organic dust—sulfur, starch, wood, flour, sugar, carbon, rubber, and some plastics are examples. When the dust reaches sufficient concentration, and its powder reaches minimum ignition energy because an ignition source is available, an explosion will take place.

The environment must be controlled to minimize the explosion potential. Hybrid explosions, due to a combination of materials in an isolated space, present an even greater danger. Each material may require extra controls when contained with other materials. The danger is when several materials are near their combustion points and join in the explosion. An example could be a low level of cornstarch being blended with iron oxide pigments. The system may be designed to safely handle the pigments, but the cornstarch will accelerate any explosion while the pigments continue to burn and limit how the system can be handled. Special design changes may be required and are dependent upon the raw materials being examined, the process, and the environment. Some possible control methods include the following:

- change the particle-size distribution from the supplier to minimize finer particles
- change the conveying system to minimize particle degradation
- the addition of a liquid spray to the dust atmosphere to agglomerate the fines, cool the powder to lower the ignition energy, minimize static build-up, and lower the oxygen level in the atmosphere
- increase the level of fines in the controlled environment to lower the oxygen level in the atmosphere to a point where an explosion cannot occur

Additional methods should be examined to minimize risks that may not be apparent during the development of a product, but that may be critical during production. Some of the raw material concerns to be aware of include the following: Explosibility Index (Kst), Minimum Ignition Energy (MIE), Minimum Ignition Temperature (MIT), Limiting Oxygen Concentration (LOC), Minimum Explosible Concentration (MEC), Volume Resistivity (Ω), Charge Decay Time, Electrostatic

Chargeability, and Self-heating Onset Temperature. The raw material supplier may be able to address these issues if specifically requested. Since non-bulk storage and dust collection are less of a concern, the information may not be automatically made available for small lots used for laboratory testing. These tests can be performed by a few outside laboratories where a one-meter sphere is used to force an explosion and measure the values. Tests run between $3000 and $5000 per ingredient or formula being tested (2012 values in the U.S.).

REFERENCES

1. Wilson, J. B. and Moore, R. J. *Harry's Cosmeticology*, 757—799, Seventh Ed., Chemical Publishing Co., 1982.
2. Oldshue, J. Y. and Herbst, N. R., *A Guide To Fluid Mixing*, 29, Mixing Equipment Company, 1990.
3. Patton, T. C., *Paint Flow and Pigment Dispersion*, 2, J. Wiley and Sons, second edition, 1979.
4. Bridgeman, P. W. *Dimensional Analysis*, New haven, Yale University Press, 1931.
5. Hoogendoorn, C. J. and den Hartog, A. P. *Chem. Eng. Sci.* , 1689, 1967, **22**.
6. Rushton, J. H., Costich, E. W. and Evrett, H. J. *Chem. Eng. Progress.* , 395, 1950, **46**.
7. Rushton, J. H., Costich, E. W. and Evrett, H. J. *Chem. Eng. Progress.* , 467, 1950, **46**.
8. Oldshue, J. Y. and Sprague, J., *Paint Varn. Prod.* , 19, 1974, **64**.
9. Oldshue, J. Y., *Fluid Mixing Technology*, 40, McGraw-Hill Publishing Company, 1983.
10. Nagata, S., Yanagimoto, M. and Tokiyama, T., *Mem. Fac.., Kyoto Univ.* , 444, 1956, 18.
11. Courtesy of Charles Ross and Son Company, Hauppauge, New York.
12. Mohr, W. D., Saton, R. L. and Jepson, C. H., *Ind. Eng. Chem.* , 1857, 1957, **49**.
13. Courtesy of Schröder and Boos Misch- und Anlagentechnik GmbH & Co. KG, Bremerhaven, Germany.
14. Courtesy of Lee® Industries, Philipsburg, Penn.
15. Courtesy of Chemineer®-Greerco® , Inc., North Andover, Mass.
16. Oldshue, J. Y., *Ind. Eng. Chem.* , 79, 1969, **61**.
17. Zweitering, T. N., *Chem. Eng. Sci.* , 244, 1958, **8**.

18. Nienow, A. W., *Chem. Eng. Sci.* , 1453, 1968, **23**.
19. Pavlushenko, I. S., *Zh. Prikl. Khim.* , 1160, 1957, **30**.
20. Oyama, Y. and Endoh, K. *Chem. Eng. (Tokyo)* , 66, 1956, **20**.
21. Weisman, J. and Efferding, L. E., *A. I. Ch. E. J.* , 419, 1960, **6**.
22. MacNeill, C., Sneeringer, J. R. and Szatmary, *A. Pharmaceutical Engineering*, 37,1985, Vol. 5 No. 6
23. London, F., Z. *Phys. Chem.* , 222, 1930, **11**.
24. Lippschitz, E., M. *Soviet Phys.* , 73, *JEPT* 1956, **2**.
25. Manegold, E., in *Kapillarsysteme.* Heidelberg, Verlag Strassenbau, Chemie und Technik, 524, 1955.
26. Rumpf, H., Strength of Granules and Agglomerates. in *Agglomeration.* Ed. Knapper, New York, Wiley 1974.

COLD-PROCESS EMULSIFICATION PRODUCING SUB-MICRON DISPERSIONS: FORMULATION AND AESTHETIC ENHANCEMENT OF COSMETIC AND OTC PRODUCTS

Authors
Michael Ross and James Wilmott
Leading Edge Innovations, LLC, 50 Tannery Road, Suite #5,
Branchburg, New Jersey 08876

ABSTRACT:

In view of the trend to reduce costs and increase convenience of emulsion preparation, especially in these days of consumer safety concerns, energy saving focus and environmental consciousness, new technologies are needed to address global concerns. One potential solution utilizes an alternate approach to formulating conventional emulsion-like products. This approach enables cosmetic scientists to prepare personal care and OTC drug products more rapidly and more reproducibly. Unlike conventional emulsions, with typical particle sizes exceeding 3 microns this process generates sub-micron, oil-in-water micelles, which are 1/10th to 1/20th the particle size of conventional emulsions.

Oils and other hydrophobic materials used in these systems have different physical and chemical properties which are distinct from conventional emulsions where the properties of both the oil and water are modified by the nature and quantity of the surface active agent(s) employed. Hydrophobic materials take on very different, desirable tactile properties when the dispersed phase particles are reduced significantly in size. The resulting sub-micron systems can be easily mixed into a rheologically modified matrix and are able to generate either conventional or highly unique tactile experiences. On a laboratory scale, the products are prepared in a single beaker so there is no need for separate sub-phases, and no heating, shearing or cooling is required! This cold-process formulation technique takes from 5 to 15 minutes per batch resulting in a significant improvement in productivity and new opportunities for unconventional product distinctions. This technique can also be readily transferred to the larger scale vessels used in the production of the final product.

TABLE OF CONTENTS

13.2.1 CONTEMPORARY COSMETICS

In the late 1960s and early 1970s functional skin treatment products emerged. Product performance expanded beyond the amelioration of superficial dryness, and their benefits evolved to a higher therapeutic level. The boundary between cosmetics and dermatological products began to blur. Cosmetic problems such as aging, uneven skin pigmentation, slack skin, cellulite, sensitive skin, oily skin, and dryness were identified and agents were sourced or developed to address these conditions. These skin disorders were often associated with conditions such as sunburn, acne, and the need for topical analgesia, etc. Cosmetics turned more to medicine for its resources, and dermatology became a source for agents that could provide either a marketing or performance advantage.

As the number and potency of functional materials increased, there arose a need to control the delivery of these agents in order to mitigate potential irritation, target their transfer to the desired location in the skin, or protect environmentally unstable materials for a commercially viable period of time. Again, the personal care market borrowed from the latest advances in medical research. *Table 1* is a summary of some of the major delivery systems currently being used in the personal care market place, the types of active they carry, and their primary benefit.

Table1: Delivery Systems Most Commonly Used in Personal Care

Classification	Description	Diameter	Materials Carried
Liposomes	Phospholipid-based unilamellar or multilamellar bilayer vessicles.	100-500 nm	Hydrophilic and hydrophobic actives
Nanodispersions	Phospholipid-based micellular dispersion.	100-500 nm	Hydrophobic actives
Vesicles	Surfactant-based vesicles or micelles	100-500 nm	Typically hydrophobic actives
Polymeric	Crosslinked acrylate or allyl methacrylate polymer	10-500 micron	Typically hydrophobic actives
Microencapsulates	Aldehyde crosslinked protein	100-5000 micron	Typically hydrophobic actives
Encapsulates	Crosslinked guar, alginate or other carbohydrate polymer	5-500 micron	Typically hydrophobic actives
Entrapment/ Clatharate	Clatharate of cyclodextrin	N/A	Hydrophobic actives
Linked	Active ingredient is covalently or ionically linked to polymeric support	N/A	Hydrophilic and hydrophobic actives

a. The Future

The trend toward even greater performance in personal care products will continue as we move further into the 21st century. New, more potent therapeutic agents are being sourced from the fields of biotechnology, pharmaceuticals, and botanicals. Materials such as enzymes, growth factors, antioxidants, cytokines, DNA, genetic promoters, epigenetic modifiers and other sophisticated materials are already being evaluated in the research facilities of leading manufacturers and suppliers. These agents, though more effective than previously used actives, are often sensitive to environmental conditions such as oxygen, heat and light. Thus, there will be a need for equally sophisticated delivery systems that will maintain or enhance the efficacy of these sensitive actives from their formulation and environmental surroundings.

While drug delivery systems have received much attention because of their potential, what is often overlooked is the vehicle into which these delivery systems are incorporated. The latter part of this chapter will focus on the proper selection of the vehicle into which the delivery systems are added, in order to ensure their performance is not compromised. The chapter will also explore a new approach to vehicle development that is complementary to most, if not all, delivery systems. This new approach is actually a true innovation in formulation science. The technology employed offers virtually unlimited aesthetic and form modification capabilities that will enable the user to truly enjoy the experience of applying the product. This new approach is called Sub-micron Micelle-Based Formulating.

b. Properties of Emulsions

Clearly, the preferred cosmetic and personal care vehicle for topical application contains both aqueous and anhydrous phases. Such products have virtually unlimited aesthetic properties and can be applied in many forms such as serums, lotions and creams. However, these components are generally incompatible with one another unless an agent is added that more significantly reduces the interfacial tension between the oil and the water phases. To do this, it is necessary to change the native properties of the oil phase and the water phase to make them more compatible with one another. This phenomenon allows the formation of a two-phase system in which one of the phases (e.g., the "oil") is suspended in the other (e.g., the water). Such ingredients are called "surface active agents" ("surfactants"). A special sub-category of surfactants is called an emulsifier. These materials not only lower the interfacial tension at the oil/water interface but, with the input of shearing energy, they enable the formation of droplets of one phase within the other. Such emulsifiers have a wide range of surface-active properties. When carefully selected, they can stabilize the incorporation of oil into a water phase or water into an oil phase. The resulting product is called an emulsion. In many cases such emulsions are prepared by heating the oil and water phases to a temperature of 70° C or greater before combining the two phases. The purpose of heating the phases is to ensure that all waxes used are melted, and that the two phases have a low enough viscosity so the two phases can mix freely. The oil and water phases are typically mixed together until they achieve a homogeneous appearance. Thereafter, they are slowly cooled to ensure the formation of appropriately small-sized droplets. It is essential that the droplets be very small in order to ensure the stability of the emulsion since, in these cases, Brownian motion will retard sedimentation. Such emulsions typically have a homogeneous, opaque, white appearance. They provide a smooth, pleasant feel upon application to the skin, hair, or other epithelial surfaces. In fact, the fields of surfactant chemistry and emulsion science have become a major disciplinary area that a competent cosmetic chemist must master in order to be a successful formulator. The proper use of surfactants to form all of the various types of useful emulsions can become a totally engaging, lifelong pursuit. The vehicle formed by the combination of an aqueous phase with an anhydrous phase will be the primary focus of the remainder of this chapter.

c. Issues with Emulsions

The introduction of surfactants to the cosmetic industry has provided a "double-edged sword" for formulators. Although the many different types of surfactants have yielded a vast array of cosmetics with very desirable aesthetic properties, the issues associated with their use have not been properly addressed. To the formulator, the development of emulsion-based products is replete with problems. Such development is a time consuming process. Further, these issues are generally limiting towards the goal of achieving desirable aesthetic properties. These issues can produce thermodynamically unstable, non-reproducible and difficult-to-scale emulsions in the manufacturing process.

It is easy to understand, therefore, why the time to develop a traditional emulsifier-based product is so lengthy. Seldom does a formulating company's Marketing department or Business Development function request exactly the same formulation. Generally, new marketing concepts will necessitate a change in composition from prior art. This change can cause a cascade of undesirable events. Different aesthetic properties are also frequently requested by Marketing in order to generate new products with new claims. When changes to either the aqueous phase or oil phase are made, the emulsifier blend, which was effective in previous systems, generally must be altered. Altering the emulsifier blend may result in a change in one or more aesthetic, performance, or safety properties. Immediate stability of the composition is often compromised as a result and, worse, such instability is not usually identified until the second or third month of accelerated stability testing. This behavior may indicate a potential problem with the long-term shelf life of the product, and it is insidious since it requires either re-balancing of the emulsifier ratios or a change in the emulsifiers selected. This has forced the industry to develop methods to predict the degree of hydrophobicity of the oil phase in order to marry it with the necessary changes to the water phase in order to permit the formation of a stable emulsion. Systems such as the HLB (Hydrophile-Lipophile Balance) have been devised. This assigns a relative numerical value to the degree of lipophilicity of a given oil, which enables the formulator to select the necessary emulsier, or blend of emulsifiers required. This approach was first developed by William Griffin who was employed by Imperial Cosmetic Industries (ICI). (1) This method has proven to be invaluable when preparing standard emulsion products. However, it becomes less predictive as the lipophilic phase becomes more complex through a mixture of soluble oils and is less relevant where blends of insoluble lipophilic agents are used.

Generally, a sequential approach to problem resolution will result in an extended time to develop a product. This will result in a delay in the projected launch date that can cost the organization millions of dollars in anticipated revenues. As a consequence, the formulator is best served by trying to anticipate potential issues. Multiple batches, having several ingredient variations, are typically prepared in order to address any unexpected contingencies. This process is filled with unnecessary redundancy and is generally unacceptable in commercial practice. Compounding the above mentioned issue is the effect that processing can have on the outcome of a batch. Emulsion stability is dependent on a variety of parameters such as the zeta potential, particle size, crystal formation, and water-binding activity (2) of the ingredients employed to achieve the desired rheological properties of the product. These parameters are dependent on the temperature to which the oil and water phases are heated, the rate of heating, the method and rate of mixing of the phases when combined at elevated temperatures, and the rate of cooling. Most emulsions require heating to insure that all higher melting point materials, such as waxes and butters, are completely melted, dissolved or dispersed in the appropriate phase.

Further, many raw materials with unique aesthetic properties cannot be emulsified easily, if at all. Useful molecular weight silicones, silicone and hydrocarbon-based gels, and fluorinated compounds are all very difficult to incorporate into a stable emulsion system.

Traditional emulsion systems also create difficulties in manufacturing. The need for heating and cooling systems, specialized high and low-shear mixing, and assorted additional processing devices makes the manufacture of emulsion systems very capital intensive. Further, the equipment specifications and energy requirements will vary from country to country. This situation will cause a modification in the processing variables thereby making it almost impossible to have a truly "global" manufacturing protocol. The energy needed to process such products can be significant and undoubtedly will add to the final cost of the finished unit. This is especially true in Europe and Asia where the price of energy is very expensive. Similarly, there is a long duration of time required to prepare a batch. It can take from 5 to 24 hours, or more, to complete the processing of emulsions depending on the batch size and number of sub-phases required. This reality requires intensive labor and energy that adds to cost to the final product.

The need for high temperature water or steam to heat the phases of the batch can cause damage to heat sensitive actives such as retinoids and proteins. Prolonged heating of certain materials can accelerate the reaction of the active agent with other components in the emulsion, or with air, if the material is oxygen sensitive. For example, the exposure of unsaturated hydrocarbons, such as vegetable oils, to air at high temperature can cause oxidation and lead to both rancidity and an undesirable color change. This is especially true where there is a growing consumer demand for products that are naturally-based from sustainable/renewable sources.

As indicated above, the complexity of the manufacturing procedure for personal care emulsions, and its dependence on many processing variables, leads to frequent quality issues. This is especially true with respect to the product's final textural and rheological properties. If any factors such as the heating, cooling or mixing rates are not carefully duplicated, the material prepared may have different properties than the preceding batches of the same product! As a result, the stability of the emulsion may vary from batch to batch.

Often, the difference of a single parameter is significant enough to cause the product to be outside the established optimum specifications. Inevitably, batches have to be either discarded or reworked. The lack of reproducibility is especially problematic when the product contains a physiologically active agent. Lack of reproducibility, due to manufacturing variations, can affect product performance and decrease consumer satisfaction. It also results in products having undesirable aesthetic properties that the user may perceive as a lack of quality. This will ultimately lead to consumer dissatisfaction, or reduced compliance in product use.

Some emulsions can be made without heating but these systems preclude the use of higher melting point materials that can add richness to the aesthetics of the final product. Further, if the rate of mixing is high, there is a chance that air can be entrapped in the emulsion. This phenomenon causes an undesirable decrease in the specific gravity of the product and an increase in product viscosity. Any variability in processing can lead to a range of undesirable rheological and textural properties. This issue can occur even if the formulation is not modified. The term "product by process" is well known in the patent art and describes this phenomenon. Often, if two or more formulators prepare the same product, the resulting compositions may vary considerably. This surprising variation can occur even though each person utilized the same lots of raw ingredients. The unsettling phenomenon occurs because it may be very difficult to exactly reproduce all of the processing parameters used to make an emulsion. If any of the processing variables is modified unexpectedly, particle-size variations may occur, or the crystalline properties of the emulsion can be compromised. *Table 2* is a chart containing the results from an experiment to determine the effect of processing on the final properties of a 5% petrolatum-containing cream. All preparations contained the same lots of ingredients. The data demonstrate that the viscosity and specific gravity can vary dramatically depending upon the processing parameters employed to make the batch.

Table 2: Petrolatum Cream (5%) - Standard Emulsion Test Results

Sample 1: Optimum Manufacturing Procedure				
Sample 2: Overheated Phases				
Sample 3: Forced Cooling				
Sample 4: Ambient Cooling				
Sample 5: Paddle mixing				
Sample 6: Rapid homogenization				
Sample 7: Underheated phases				
Sample	*Specific Gravity*	*Initial Viscosity (cP)*	*Viscosity (cP) 24 Hr @ 25oC*	*Viscosity (cP) 24 Hr. @ 50oC*
1	0.912	99,970	140,580	26,560
2	0.937	85,910	93,720	29,690
3	0.952	93,720	109,340	29,700
4	0.941	51,550	96,840	131,200
5	0.959	62,480	85,910	78,100
6	0.803	112,460	124,960	20,620
7	0.931	51,550	96,840	20,600
Note: Viscosity measurements were taken with a Brookfield LVT model viscometer				

Since there is so much uncertainty at the "bench" level in the laboratory, there is often concern that a typical 500-g to 2000-g lab preparation will not translate directly to a manufacturing environment. This concern is often well founded. Compounding this scale-up problem is the fact that equipment used in the laboratory generally does not correlate with that used in the plant. There is usually a need for an intermediate phase during scale-up that facilitates this transition. Some equipment is engineered to mimic plant conditions but at a fraction of the size. Even so, scale-up issues abound. To deal with the vagaries of scale-up, the product may be subjected to a wide range of processing variations in order to optimize the conditions of manufacture. Products made at each level of scale-up are typically subjected to accelerated stability testing in order to ensure the integrity of the product for its anticipated shelf- life. When one adds the processing variability and the need for scale up to the uncertainty of the selection of the emulsifier system, it is almost a wonder that any product ever makes it to the market on time. As a consequence, most formulators tend to stay with the tried and true approaches of the past. A significant alteration to these systems or the development of an entirely new system is often laced with unknown issues that can severely jeopardize the introduction of a new product.

13.2.2 FACTORS DRIVING THE SEARCH FOR ALTERNATE APPROACHES

The current practices for making emulsified formulations have a number of limitations in their use. The main factors are 1) the difficulty in creating new aesthetic and textural experiences; 2) the issue of delivering the sophisticated physiologically active agents to enhance product efficacy; 3) Marketplace confusion; 4) the expansion of regulatory restrictions; 5) the desire to utilize more natural and sustainable materials.

a. Textural Diversity

Current formulation practices have produced a number of unique products with a variety of textural properties, however, it is becoming increasingly more difficult to satisfy the current market demand for new approaches to expand the experiential elements and maximize performance. The traditional approach has been to create different types of surfactants and emulsifying agents, but these have generally produced different ways of providing a similar effect. Today's market is demanding more than the minimalistic change being provided by the current formulating paradigm. It is seeking dramatic effects, not subtle nuances.

b. Enhanced Performance

Because the use of emulsifiers and other surface-active agents changes the physical and chemical properties of the oil and water phases to permit emulsification, they also modify the beneficial properties of the hydrophilic and lipophilic functional ingredients added to the composition to deliver product performance. As a result, usually only modest improvement in skin condition, wear properties, fragrance impression, cleansing efficacy, etc. can be realized. Ironically, the very agents that permit the formation of viable oil-in-water or water-in-oil micelles may be responsible for the suppression of product performance. Further, the environment produced is hostile to liposomes and other delivery vehicles that could help maximize the active ingredient's benefit.

c. Marketplace Confusion

The proliferation of marketed products that have seemingly contradictory positions is creating consumer confusion. As a consequence, consumers have taken it upon themselves to learn more about the products that they are using. They are becoming more product savvy and want to know more about the chemicals to which they are being exposed. While much of this information is useful, some of it is either incomplete or inaccurate. Unfortunately, this has not stopped the propagation of Internet sites advocating a particular position.

d. Regulatory

Expanding consumer knowledge about products is causing the general population to pressure regulatory agencies to take action in order to maintain or preserve the safety and environmental compatibility of the materials that they are applying to their skin. Consumers are banding together to influence organizations and lobbyists in this area, which has resulted in an increase in the number of regulations that have been directing the cosmetics industry. This, in conjunction with the pressure from regulations abroad, has complicated the formulating environment to develop products that are universally acceptable.

Some of the more important regulatory factors are; the EU Directives, REACH, The Cosmetic Act of 2010, Japanese ingredient restrictions, Proposition 65, The California Green Chemistry Initiative (3), increased oversight by the FDA as well as emerging Chinese regulatory policy. While many of these legislations have similarities in their restrictions, they continue to remove materials from use and differ enough in scope that it becomes difficult to create "Globally Acceptable" formulations.

To compound the problem of globally formulating, these evolving regulations make it virtually impossible from an economic perspective, to introduce new, technologically advanced reagents into the industry. The amount of data that is required for new products to be allowed into the marketplace becomes prohibitively expensive to obtain, and causes stagnation in both product performance and aesthetics. Combined with the continuous removal of available cosmetic reagents from the positive lists, formulators are being forced to find new and unique uses for older, less controversial materials.

e. Resource Availability and Sustainability

The availability of resources and the sustainability of materials that are used in formulations has become increasingly important in recent years. There is a growing concern about the impact of synthetic chemicals on consumer health, and they are embracing the use of natural materials for their perceived nutritional and functional benefits. However, these materials require special handling to maintain their integrity. Further, natural materials are subject to shortages and unexpected price increases, which may require rapid reformulation.

Even raw materials that are in abundance have become more expensive to obtain, as the costs of energy have consistently increased and have been added on to the price tag. In fact, traditional materials that were once abundant and used ubiquitously in the marketplace, are now being replaced by less expensive, more sustainable options.

The production of conventional emulsion systems requires a tremendous amount of energy input. The entire process may rely upon extensive heating, mixing or cooling when combining raw materials into finished formulations. Unfortunately, the demand and costs of energy are increasing, which are being passed along to the consumer in the form of a more expensive product.

These and other factors have been a driving force in the search for alternate approaches to the current formulating and manufacturing paradigms.

13.2.3 SUB-MICRON MICELLES

There are alternatives to the traditional emulsification process. One of these is the formation of products utilizing the unique properties of micelles with a small particle size. Sub-micron micelles can be made with virtually any hydrophobic material by carefully controlling the selection of sub-micron production and the processing conditions during manufacture. Since the micelles of each hydrophobic material are made the same way, they are less dependent on the type of emulsifier or surfactant used, or lack thereof, and because they have approximately the same small particle size, there is much less tendency for the micelles to coalesce. This phenomenon is explained by Stokes' Law, which is illustrated in an equation relating the terminal settling or rising velocity of a smooth sphere in a viscous fluid of known density and viscosity to the diameter of the sphere when subjected to a known force field (*Table 3*). Using this equation, with all other factors being constant, a 200 nm hydrophobic agent particle has a velocity of fall that is 680 times slower than one of identical composition having a 5-micron particle size of a standard emulsion.

Further, depending upon the method of manufacture, field strength/zeta potential interactions increase the propensity of the particles to repel one another. Zeta potential is a measure of the magnitude of the electrostatic or charge repulsion or attraction between particles, and is one of the fundamental parameters known to affect stability. Its measurement brings detailed insight into the causes of dispersion, aggregation or flocculation, and can be applied to improve the formulation of dispersions, emulsions and suspensions. Therefore, there is a greater desire to keep the particles apart, rather than coalesce. (4)

Additionally, the small particle size and field effect permit lipophilic phase concentrations of up to 60% w/w or more, without the high viscosity that is typically obtained when the particle size is larger. As a result, a concentrated sub-micron system will rapidly disperse into water, thereby spontaneously expanding to fill the volume of the vessel in which the water is contained. The micelles will remain in this configuration indefinitely, unless acted upon by an outside force that destabilizes the system. Further, micelle systems with separate lipophilic materials can be freely interspersed and will mutually coexist. Additionally, depending on the method of manufacture, the particle-size distribution can be very tight when properly controlled. In practice, the smaller the particle, the greater the potential benefit.

a. Benefits of Being Smaller

Small particles have a series of benefits depending on their size and uniformity. One interesting property of these systems is that they can alter the aesthetic properties of virtually all materials. This feature results in the opportunity to create new sensations with familiar lipophilic ingredients. Conventional materials such as petrolatum, lanolin, waxes and natural oils are given a new "life" and purpose. Further, the aesthetic properties can be adjusted by simply mixing lipophilic systems with different aesthetic properties to create a new and unique textural experience.

Independent of the method employed to create the sub-micron micelles, manufactured concentrates of various low polarity lipophilic agents (lipophiles) mix together readily, without issue. The practice of balancing the hydrophilic and lipophilic emulsifiers (HLB) depending on the composition of the lipophilic phase that is used so commonly in the preparation of standard supra-micron emulsion systems is now rendered insignificant. Thus, a virtually infinite array of lipophilic dispersions can be mixed, in any proportions, without creating any instability in the final blend.

The combination of individual systems of lipophilic micelles can be performed without the need of any extraordinary processing conditions. This attribute permits the rapid formulation of compositions with the desired aesthetic and performance properties. When it is applied to manufacturing, a significant reduction in both the processing time and the utilization of energy is achieved. A further explanation of these benefits will be covered in subsequent sections.

Systems of sub-micron micelles also have regulatory benefits. Since their particles size is greater than 100nm, they do not fall under the current regulatory definitions of nanotechnology, which is presently being subjected to consumer concerns and legislative action regarding their impact on health and the environment.

Table 3. Stokes' Law
• An equation relating the terminal settling or rising velocity of a smooth sphere in a viscous fluid of known density and viscosity to the diameter of the sphere when subjected to a known force field.
$V = (2gr^2)(d1\text{-}d2)/9\mu$
• V = velocity of fall (cm sec^{-1}), g = acceleration of gravity (cm sec^{-2}), r = "equivalent" radius of particle (cm), dl = density of particle (g cm^{-3}), d2 = density of medium (g cm^{-3}), and μ = viscosity of medium (dyne sec cm^{-2}).
• **200 nm particle is 680 times more stable than 5 μ particle of standard emulsion.**

13.2.4 METHODS OF PRODUCING SUB-MICRON MICELLES

There are many methods of producing sub-micron micelles. Some of the more commonly practiced methods are sonication, precipitation, high-pressure/high shear, stirred-kettle, freeze-drying, extrusion, and high surfactant loading with high-shear exposure. Any of these methods are suitable for the creation of sub-micron micelles to be used in the formulation of finished products.

Sonication can be used to create sub-micron micelles through the use of a high-energy probe that transfers its energy to the sample, and breaks up the sample into smaller and smaller particles. Sonication can be direct, applying the probe directly to the sample; or can be indirect, which would transfer the initial burst of energy into an ultrasonic bath, and then the sample would be immersed into this bath to receive the energy and break up the particles.

Precipitation is another method that may be employed to create sub-micron micelles. The hydrophobic phase is dissolved in an organic solvent and a water-soluble surfactant is dissolved in water. These two solutions are mixed and an emulsion is formed into small droplets in the aqueous phase. The water-soluble surfactant decreases the tension at the interphase between the water and the organic solution, allows emulsification to take place, and stabilizes the droplets formed against aggregation or coalescence. The final step involves removal of the organic solvent by evaporation. The hydrophobic phase precipitates and one particle is formed from each droplet. A suspension of small spherical hydrophobic particles is formed. The particle size is dependent upon the surfactant concentration and on the emulsification energy imparted.

High-Pressure/High Shear can be used to create sub-micron micelles as well. This methodology combines a hydrophilic and a lipophilic phase with the help of a facilitating agent and then processes them together at pressures between 5,000 and 50,000psi. Facilitating agents may include any class of surfactant or emulsifier. Generally, lower amounts of surfactant or emulsifier are required when pursuing this method of sub-micron micelle creation.

In freeze-drying, two available methods are thin film freezing and spray freeze-drying. In spray freeze-drying, for example, an aqueous solution containing active ingredients is atomized into the cold gas above a cryogenic liquid. The atomized particles adsorb onto the gas-liquid interface and aggregate there as sub-micron micelles.

Sub-micron micelles can also be created using high surfactant loadings in combination with high shear. In these cases, an appropriate surfactant is used at an atypically high level, in combination with high shear mixing. The method of imparting high shear is unimportant, and resulting particles can vary in size, but are below 1000nm.

13.2.5 FORMULATING WITH SUB-MICRON MICELLES

Traditional methods of formulating products rely on a multitude of factors in order to achieve success. These traditional systems require the separation of lipophilic and hydrophilic phases, the selection of an appropriate surfactant/emulsifier, an extended period of high temperature/high energy processing, and then an extended period of cooling/force-cooling under specific processing conditions. Each of these steps create an opportunity for mistakes and promotes an environment that is rife with variability. Formulating with sub-micron micelles removes many of the troublesome steps in formulation.

Formulations using sub-micron micelles utilize cold-process conditions. Lipophilic and hydrophilic phases are pre-formed into high concentration sub-phases, where they are incorporated together to form finished formulations. The need for high temperature exposure and high energy processing is removed, and the consistency between batches is increased substantially.

Perhaps one of the greatest benefits of formulating with sub-micron micelles, is the speed at which formulations can be created. Without the heating and specialized processing requirements of traditional formulations, several modifications of an existing formulation can be prepared within a very short period of time. This allows the formulator to quickly perform range-finding techniques when working to match a new benchmark. The increased productivity reduces the time needed to get to a final marketed product.

Another benefit of sub-micron micelles is their formulating flexibility. All sub-micron concentrates are compatible with each other. Normally the combination of incompatible lipophilic materials can present a daunting challenge to the formulation when using standard emulsification processes, the separate formation of lipophilic sub-micron systems can be readily mixed without the concern of instability. Such classes as silicones, hydrocarbons, natural oils, alkyl esters, fragrances, waxes, butters, fluorocarbons, and other lipophilic agents can be combined without issue.

Although traditional formulations require rebalancing of HLB when additional hydrophobes are incorporated into the formulation, this is not necessary when working with sub-micron micelles. Sub-micron micelle concentrates are highly compatible with each other. When the particles are made small, concepts such as HLB become far less consequential, and materials that are typically unable to be combined, are suddenly compatible.

One of the biggest problems faced by formulators is the need to deliver unique aesthetics in their new products. This task has become increasingly difficult as regulatory pressures and companies' internal negative lists grow on an almost daily basis. The ability to mix and match highly concentrated sub-micron micelles with one another allows for a virtually limitless variety of unique aesthetic properties. Since each lipophilic sub-micron micelle system has a different aesthetic profile they can be blended to achieve an intermediate aesthetic experience. In fact, having sub-micron micelle systems of just 13 materials with different aesthetic properties permits the formation of a 13 (6.227×10^9) factorial number of possibility of different aesthetic benefits which represents a potentially different aesthetic experience for everyone in the world.

Concentrated dispersions of sub-micron micelles can be prepared and then characterized by their aesthetic, tactile and rub-in qualities. When prepared in this method, the dispersions can be assigned semi-quantitative values that correspond to their characteristics. A numerical value may be assigned from 1 to 1000 or some iteration thereof. With the numbers corresponding to specific characteristics, the combination of sub-micron concentrates can be meaningfully used to alter the final aesthetics of finished formulations, and their complete compatibility allows for limitless combinations, creating unique finished formulations.

Given all of the aforementioned benefits, the resulting formulations have incredible consistency. Without the variation in particle size that is typical of traditional formulations, products made with sub-micron micelles impart consistent and predictable aesthetics into the finished formulation each time. A suitable rheological modifier is added to the water phase and adjusts for viscosity and texture, then the sub-micron micelle systems are added with minimal agitation to complete the formulation.

The challenge of transferring the laboratory preparation and processing procedure into a manufacturing environment can often be very difficult with a traditional emulsion approach. This is because the engineering properties of the equipment in the laboratory often are not the same as engineering properties of the equipment used in manufacturing. Thus the particle size and stability of a standard emulsion can vary tremendously between the laboratory and manufacturing. Therefore it is often necessary to change the processing conditions in manufacturing to achieve an analogous product to one made in the lab. This can often require an additional Process Development step to optimize. Thus, in standard emulsification situations the process is equally as important as the formula. However, since the process of producing separate lipophilic sub-micron micelles imparts so much energy in producing the fine particle size, they can be combined readily without the need of sophisticated shearing and heat transfer equipment. The use of sub-micron micelles makes the transfer from the laboratory to manufacturing a rudimentary task.

13.2.6 MANUFACTURING BENEFITS

Sub-micron micellular formulations have distinct advantages in the manufacturing area. Without the need for extended periods of heating, the ingredients of the formulation remain intact and are not subjected to any degradation due to excessive heat exposure. The process conditions are uncomplicated. They are significantly less expensive to produce, and without the need for sophisticated manufacturing equipment and/or conditions, can be successfully and reproducibly made anywhere in the world.

a. Protection of Key Materials

Manufacturing with sub-micron micelles employs a cold-process technique. Removing extended heating steps from the formulation allows for more confident use of sensitive materials in the product. The risk of promoting oxidation or degradation of these materials is completely removed, and results in a more pristine manufactured product.

b. Consistency and Reproducibility

Formulations made with sub-micron micelles are often far more simple to compound and do not require as many separate ingredients as their traditional counterparts. There are few if any critical steps in the manufacturing process that could affect the outcome of the final product. Thus they are less "compounder dependent". There are typically fewer materials to incorporate into the batch, and there are no separate oil and water phases which must be heated, combined and properly sheared to produce the final emulsion. Quality is dramatically improved since it is much easier to ensure batch-to-batch reproducibility. There is little waste, and virtually no "rework" of a batch is required. Thus, it eliminates the cost associated with reworking, salvaging, and disposing of out-of specification product as well as avoids the cost of lost opportunity while personnel/equipment are tied up in the salvage operation.

c. Reduced Manufacturing Cost

Labor, overhead, and processing time can be reduced from 50 to 75%. This improvement in production efficiency results in plant capacity increases without any additional capital investment. If capital equipment is needed, it will generate savings of about 70 to 80% as compared to processing equipment needed for the manufacture of conventional emulsions. Since neither heating nor cooling is required, energy savings can be greater than 90%. Kettle dwell time is greatly reduced, and the product can be transferred directly to the filling line once ingredient additions are completed. In fact, continuous processing is possible. A summary of the cost savings that can be realized when manufacturing with sub-micron micelles is found in *Table 4* below.

Table 4: Summary of Manufacturing Benefits

Energy Savings	> 90%
Capital Savings	> 70%
Overhead Savings	> 50%
Process Time Reduction	> 50%
Efficiency Enhancement	> 50%
Revenue Improvement	> 100%
Earnings Improvement	> 100%
Margin Improvement	1–3%
Capital Savings	> 70%

d. Global Consistency

Finally, the ease of manufacturing enables the product made with sub-micron micelles to be made exactly the same in any location in the world. This allows companies the flexibility to transfer production to their manufacturing plant of choice, and potentially save resources that would otherwise have been exhausted on import and export.

13.2.7 CONSUMER BENEFITS

The use of sub-micron micelles in the formulation of cosmetics and OTC products has many benefits to the consumer. Some of these include: improved product efficacy, unique aesthetic properties, reduced environmental impact, consistent quality, and greater consumer safety.

While consumers continue to demand more and more from their products from an experiential as well as a quality standpoint and performance perspective; continuously increasing regulatory constraints have tempered innovation and tied the hands of the formulators' abilities to deliver on these desires. Through the use of sub-micron micelles in the formulation of products, the limitations of current practices are lifted, and a new conduit to unique and effective formulations is created.

The availability of detailed information about cosmetics and the chemicals that they are comprised of has given rise to changes in both consumer perceptions and expectations. The new face of the consumer can be seen through the multitude of activists, bloggers, press and beauty websites.

a. Enhanced Product Efficacy

Consumers would also benefit from an increase in product performance, associated with the use of sub-micron micelles. This performance enhancement is due to an increase of surface area, resulting in a greater diffusion of functional agents into the skin. The reduction or elimination of emulsifiers may permit the use of advanced delivery systems that can both facilitate the movement of the active ingredients into the skin and protect them from the harsh environmental conditions that can deactivate their benefits. Additionally, the cold-process conditions used to make the individual micelle systems and their ultimate assembly into a final product does not expose the functional agents to the severe high-temperature processing conditions of standard emulsions. With less surface-active agents required in the formulations, the potential for active ingredients to become denatured or otherwise diminished in their activity is greatly reduced.

b. Unique Aesthetic Experiences

Small particles provide a new tactile experience to the same, commonly used reagents in the laboratory. Formulations can have the same ingredient listing on the package, yet feel significantly different when applied to the skin. This phenomenon relates to the increased packing capacity of the particles, while avoiding the increased viscosity and undesirable tactile properties of a standard emulsion of the same composition. The consumer has the additional benefit of having higher levels of hydrophobic actives and other ingredients loaded into their products without sacrificing the experience.

c. Consistency and Reproducibility

In accordance with Stokes' Law, the rate of creaming or sedimentation becomes exponentially slower as the particle size is decreased, and consequently, the more stable the suspension becomes. The lipophilic materials are processed in a manner to create a particle-size distribution that is extremely narrow. These systems can be readily mixed in the final composition to produce a consistent, highly reproducible product. The consumer experiences the same benefits with each use or with each new product purchased. In the case of purchasing products that have been formulated with sub-micron micelles, the consumer is benefitted with a more stable formulation that would require fewer ancillary stabilizing agents in comparison to the traditionally formulated products in the marketplace. This reduction in stabilizing agents promotes shorter ingredient lists, leading to a less intimidating experience for consumers when comparing products.

Another important benefit for consumers is quality and consistency. Traditional formulations require excessive heating/cooling and shearing conditions in order to successfully be produced. During the heating phase, there is a strong propensity for the systems to lose water, as hot water vapor escapes the production vessel. Additionally, during the emulsification phase of production, simply combining the oil and water phase at a rate of addition that is either too fast or too slow, can alter the results of the end-product. In addition to these caveats, the product must be cooled down to room temperature, while adding other materials to complete the batch. It is during this cool-down process that there is further potential for problems; such as cooling down too quickly, not cooling down quickly enough, shearing too much and shearing too little. All of these steps in the manufacturing process can lead to highly variable particle sizes of the emulsion, variable product aesthetics and a high level of inconsistency between batches.

Products formulated with sub-micron micelles are not reliant upon the same conditions as traditional products. Prior to compounding a finished product, sub-micron micelles are formed through one of the commercially available methods to have a uniform particle size with a very narrow distribution. Once accepted, these particles are simply combined into the finished formulation under ambient conditions, and mixed until uniform. There are no special processing procedures required at the time of compounding the finished formulation, and the resulting product is of high quality with exceptional reproducibility. With this simplified process, consumers are able to obtain the same product from anywhere in the world, and anytime they purchase the product.

d. Safety

While products created with sub-micron micelles are elegant and more aesthetically pleasing, some methods of producing these small particles allow for the ability to use fewer/lower levels of surface active agents. This is important to consumers that have sensitive skin, as these formulations tend to be far less irritating than their traditional counterparts.

e. Environmental

Consumers are becoming more cognizant of the need to use more sustainable materials and minimize the impact of their actions on the environment. One of the most relevant, yet unseen benefits for consumers is the fact that formulations created using sub-micron micelles are more environmentally friendly than their traditional counterparts. They can make elegant products out of sustainable, natural materials because they have pleasant textural properties. Further, the environmental impact can be minimized because, while there are many methods of producing sub-micron micelles, most of these methods result in far less energy consumption than standard products. In many cases, these products can be created completely by cold-processing conditions without the need for excessive heating and cooling during the creation of these products. As a result, their carbon footprint, energy consumption, and use of resources are significantly reduced.

CONCLUSION

Lipophilic sub-micron micelles offer many advantages versus the conventional approach to making traditional emulsifier-based cosmetic, personal care, and drug products. They can be prepared using various techniques, but all share the benefits associated with their smaller size. Unlike conventional emulsions, with typical particle sizes exceeding 3 microns, sub-micron oil-in-water micelles are 1/10th to 1/20th the particle size of conventional emulsions. They provide new properties to existing lipophilic materials, enhance product efficacy, and offer many consumer, manufacturing, and formulating benefits. This approach enables cosmetic scientists and process engineers to prepare personal care and OTC drug products more rapidly and more reproducibly. It addresses many of the regulatory and financial concerns that are associated with current practices. The compatibility of sub-micron micelle systems with delivery systems and new, emerging, therapeutic agents makes this technology an ideal formulating vehicle. The novel technical approach provided by the use of sub-micron micelles opens the door for a whole new range of possibilities for today's cosmetic chemist and end user.

REFERENCES

1. The HLB System a time-saving guide to emulsifier selection edited and reprinted from Chemmunique, publication of ICI Americas Inc. ICI Americas Inc. Wilmington, Delaware 19897 Anticipating Needs
2. Zeta Potential: An Introduction in 30 Minutes; Latin American Journal of Pharmacy (formerly Acta Farmacéutica Bonaerense) Lat. Am. J. Pharm.28 (2): 313-7 (2009) Note to the EditorReceived: January 13, 2009Accepted: January 17, 2009 The Studies on Hydrophilic-Lipophilic Balance (HLB): Sixty Yearsafter William C. Griffin's Pioneer Work (1949-2009) Ricardo C. Pasquali *, Natalia Sacco & Carlos Brengi Cátedra de Farmacotecnia I, Departamento de Tecnología Farmacéutica, Facultad de Farmacia y Bioquímica, Universidad de Buenos Aires, Junín 956, 6° piso (1113) Buenos Aires, Argentina
3. The California Green Chemistry Initiative (http://www.dtsc.ca.gov/PollutionPrevention/GreenChemistryInitiative/)
4. Suspension stability: Why particle size, zeta potential and rheology are important; Dr John Duffy/Dr Adrian Hill Product Technical Specialists Rheometry Products Malvern Instruments Limited

INTELLIGENT SELECTION AND MANUFACTURE OF NATURAL EXTRACTS

Author
Satish Nayak, PhD
Kemin Industries,
2100 Maury Street, Des Moines, Iowa – 50317, USA.

ABSTRACT

Consumers and ingredient suppliers are both concerned about the *quality of personal care products* used on the hair, face, and body. In today's Internet-connected world, consumers want to know the *source of the ingredients* that are being used in the manufacture of their cosmetic and personal care products. Ingredient suppliers understand that the products containing ingredients derived from plants have more consumer appeal, and are viewed by them as being safer than those obtained synthetically.

In response to this consumer trend, many personal care products are being launched that contain natural extracts. These provide a wide variety of benefits to the user, and have claims such as being anti-inflammatory, antioxidants, skin whiteners, skin firming, etc. For these natural extracts to be successful, it is important to understand the key active molecule, or a group of molecules, responsible for the observed effect in the specified application. It is furthermore important that the right plant source and extraction method is chosen for the extraction of these actives in order to ensure that natural extracts are produced at a reasonable cost.

This chapter provides several examples of selection of the right plant source, for a variety of actives and different manufacturing processes in order to be used to produce a safe, consistent, and efficacious natural extract.

TABLE OF CONTENTS

13.3.1 INTRODUCTION

The trend for using natural products is ever increasing, primarily due to the consumer perception that natural ingredients are safe. To accommodate this consumer perception, the same trend is mirrored in product labels that claim to have natural or nature-derived ingredients. Ingredient suppliers are now focusing more on supplying natural and plant or bio-based products. The functionality of these ingredients spans a wide range from antioxidants to antimicrobials to emulsifiers. The active molecules to which these functionalities have been attributed tend to be produced in small quantities in their parent sources. Also, the complexity that Mother Nature has incorporated in these molecules makes their synthetic production economically unfeasible. Hence choosing the right source and the extraction technique plays a vital role in the optimal functionality of these ingredients in a cosmetics formulation.

Traditionally, the active components from plants or other biological sources have been extracted by using water or hydrocarbon solvents. Along with the objection of having residual solvents in the extracts as well as recent advancements in analytical and physical chemistry, several sophisticated extraction techniques have been developed. These techniques have substantially improved the extraction yields, reduced the usage of organic solvents, and reduced the time and investment that is needed to introduce commercially viable natural extracts in the market. There are several factors that need to be taken into account before choosing the right extraction technique.

- **Target Molecule** – The chemical properties of the active compound or the class of compound to be extracted. Primarily polarity and molecular weight, if known.
- **Source** – The source of the active molecule; plant, algae, microbes. Also the ability of the source to accumulate the desired molecule and any potential of impurities or nondesired molecules that might interfere with the extraction.
- **Regulatory/Certifications** – The natural certification or the regulatory approval that is desired for the obtained extract. Many extraction techniques and solvents are on the not-allowed list of regulatory and certification agencies. The list is not universal but is region-specific to the intended geographical market for the extract.
- **Efficacy** – The chosen extraction technique should not affect the efficacy of the desired molecule by degrading it or making it inactive during the extraction process.

The primary aim of this chapter is to give readers a general overview of the principles and abilities of different extraction technologies for extracting actives from natural sources. Some of the techniques discussed are Microwave Assisted Extraction (MAE), Ultrasonic Assisted Extraction (UAE), and Supercritical Fluid Extraction (SCFE). In addition to the extraction techniques, consideration should be given to the natural sources for the active molecules, which can have a major impact on the commercial value of an extract. Most often the activity of an extract could be attributed to a combination of molecules rather than a single molecule. The amount of complexity and redundancy that Mother Nature imparts to a particular functionality, such as antioxidants or antimicrobials, is immense. Usually it is more than one molecule that is responsible for these functionalities, and care should be taken that the majority of the molecules from that group are extracted for the resulting extract to provide "complete" functionality.

13.3.2 SOURCES OF NATURAL INGREDIENTS

Natural actives can be obtained from variety of sources. Since there is no firm legal definition for natural ingredients, many animal-based ingredients could also be considered as natural. This chapter focuses only on non-animal-based sources.

a. Plants

Medicinal disciplines such as Ayurveda, Yunani, and Traditional Chinese Medicines have developed practices that rely heavily on plant-based ingredients for curing various ailments. It is a common belief among all the traditional medicinal practices that Mother Nature provides solutions to all the health problems. Most of these practices are based on empirical evidence and trial and error. It is only recently, due to advances in various scientific disciplines, we have started to understand the active compounds that are the cause for such benefits. For example, it was always known that eating green leafy vegetables such as broccoli, kale, and spinach was beneficial to the eyes. It was only recently, when these vegetables were analyzed, it was found that they were high in carotenoids such as lutein and zeaxanthin that contribute to eye health. [1] In Ayurveda, turmeric is used extensively as an anti-inflammatory and antiseptic. By analyzing the turmeric root extracts this efficacy has been attributed to a class of compound called curcuminoids. [2] [3]

Plants produce a variety of phytochemicals such as terpenes, polyphenols, lipids, organic acids, protein inhibitors, etc. These phytochemicals have variety of functionalities such as being antimicrobials, antioxidants, anti-inflammatory, and thermogenic. [4] These phytochemicals are secondary metabolites that are produced by plants for a variety of internal functions. Their production is highly dependent on the season, environmental conditions, and age of the plant. [5] [6] The choice of the right plant for extracting a certain active is crucial to the commercial viability of that extract. Several factors such as the application of the extract, market value, yield of the active on per acre basis, and extraction technology need to be taken into account.

b. Microorganisms

Microorganisms have been a source of a variety of ingredients used in foods and personal care. Both bacteria and fungi have been used to produce these ingredients. One of the most common ingredients used in cosmetics produced by fermentation is citric acid. Citric acid is also produced by extracting from citrus fruits, but this process is substantially more expensive than fermentation. In the fermentation process, *Aspergillus niger* cultures are fed on glucose or sucrose obtained from natural sources that then metabolize the sugars to produce citric acid. The obtained citric acid is then extracted from the media by using an acid and a base. [7] Similarly, *Lactobacillus* strains are used in production of lactic acid, [8] which is widely known to have several skin benefits. [9] Ingredients produced by microbes have a wide range of functionalities such as antimicrobial, flavors, emulsifiers, thickeners, or surfactants. Biosurfactants such as rhamnolipids and sphorolipids have been produced by fermentation of *Pseudomonas aeruginosa* and *Candida bomicola*, respectively. [10]

Choosing an appropriate microbial strain that can produce high yields of the desired molecule is crucial for production using fermentation. Subsequent downstream processing, to separate the actives from the broth, may involve cell separation and concentration of the extract followed by precipitation or drying of the broth on a carrier or extraction by using an organic solvent.

c. Algae

In the past decade, interest in algae as a source of novel natural compounds has been growing rapidly. Algae of many types floating on the oceans are common in various regions of the world. Some of the most common ingredients extracted from algae are alginates, carrageenan, and agar, which are used for thickening and emulsifying formulations. [11] Algae have also been found to have molecules with diverse biological activities such as being antioxidant, antimicrobial, and antiviral. [12] It is understood that many of these algae live in extreme conditions and must adapt to their environment. The result of such adaptation is production of secondary metabolites that can participate in the natural defense of these organisms, which can lead to formation of complex and diverse molecules. [11] Figure 1 illustrates some of the novel molecules that are found in algae. Mycosporine glycine belongs to a class of compounds called Mycosporine-like amino acids, which have antioxidant ability. [11] Eckol belongs to class of compounds called phlorotannins, which are also antioxidants and have photoprotective effect. [11] Fucoxanthin is a xanthophyll and has been found to promote fat burning in adipose tissues. [13]

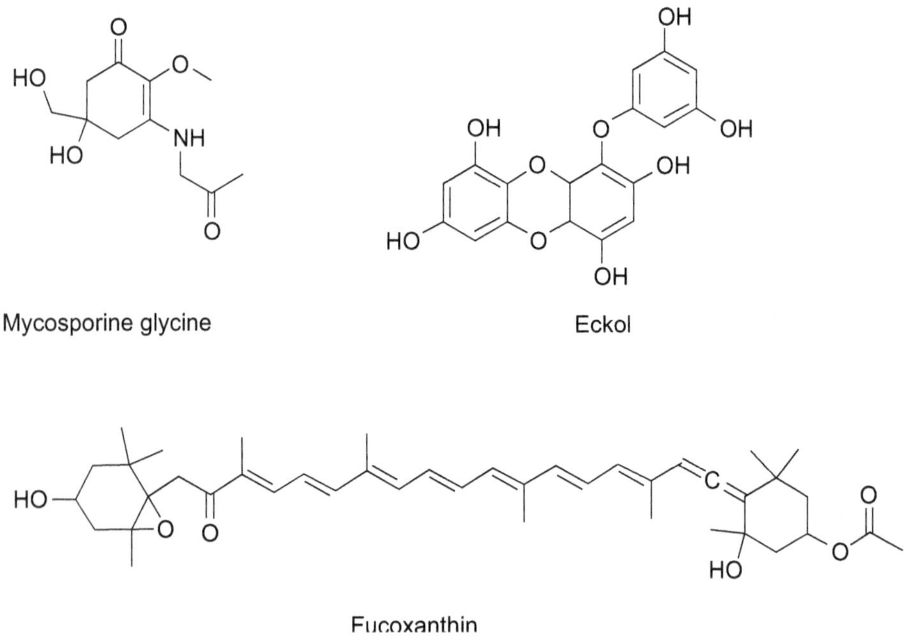

Figure 1. Structures of unique molecules found in algae.

The process of extracting molecules of interest from algae involves the following steps; algal strain development and cultivation followed by harvesting the biomass through separation and downstream processing, which may involve dewatering, extraction, fractionation, and drying. [14]

It is important that the natural source used for extraction is consistent on a batch-to-batch basis. Drastic changes in the level of actives in the source can have unfavorable impact on the subsequent extraction method and hence can affect the quality and cost of the extract. Large genetic variation in the source can lead to accumulation of varying amounts of actives that may produce extracts with different efficacies. Hence it is important to have a good control on both the species of the source and the conditions in which they are allowed to hyper-accumulate the desired actives. Such control could be obtained, for example, by cultivating a single genetic strain of the source (plant, microbial, or algal). Several natural breeding and selection techniques can be used to obtain hyper-accumulating strains that can then be propagated and grown at industrial scale. Going into details of such technologies is beyond the scope of this chapter, and readers are encouraged to read the following references. [15] [16]

13.3.3 EXTRACTION TECHNOLOGIES

Choosing the right extraction technology is as important as choosing the right natural source for a bioactive. The extraction method can have a profound effect on the endproduct that is used in the cosmetic and personal care formulations. If a sub-optimal extraction technology is used, it can result into products that are difficult to formulate. This may be due to color, odor, or impurities that are co-extracted in the process. The following section will discuss the basics of several conventional and modern extraction technologies.

a. Conventional Solvent Extraction

Solvent extraction is the most traditional and most commonly used extraction technique for separating actives from a biomass. [17] In this method, biomass is exposed to different solvents individually or to a mix of solvents depending on the desired polarity. This technology is based on the fundamental principle of "Like dissolves like," where the polarity of the extracting solvent is closely matched to that of the target molecule or a class of molecules. Most often temperature, pressure, and pH can be tuned to optimize the yields of the extract. Once the target species is extracted into the solvent phase, the spent biomass is then separated by separating technologies like centrifugation or filtration. The obtained enriched solvent can then be used directly as is, as long as the solvent employed has no toxicity associated with it. If there is toxicity associated with the used solvent then it is removed by distillation or precipitation of the target molecule.

Traditional solvent extractions have been carried out using organic solvents such as hexane, ether, dichloromethane, chloroform, and ethanol. [18] They have been used for extracting actives with different polarities; nonpolar, mid-polar, and polar. Most of these solvents have toxicity associated with them, hence they need to be removed to an acceptable level before the extract is used in the endproduct. [19] The choice of solvent will also depend on the regulatory restrictions imposed on the application of the extract. Solvent extraction may be advantageous due to the low processing cost, but the use of toxic solvents that requires their removal, most often by heat, can result in degradation of the active molecule.

Solvent-extraction techniques have been improved immensely in recent years, and have been made more efficient by use of less solvent, recycling of solvents, and concomitant use of heat and pressure during the extraction phase. All of these improvements contribute to higher yield of extraction, which in turn decreases the cost of the extract. [20] However, none of these improvements change the consumer perception about solvent-processed ingredients. The more well-informed consumers of today, relying on the Internet and social media, are more aware of the source and processing of the ingredients used in their product, and they demand that eco-friendly processes be used in the production of ingredients. This trend has led to an increase in the use of more efficient and improved modern extraction technologies for natural ingredients.

b. Microwave Assisted Extraction (MAE)

Microwaves have been applied in many fields such as: communication, navigation, astronomy, spectroscopy, and heating. [21] For extraction purposes, it is the heating aspect of microwaves that is used. In the electromagnetic spectrum, microwaves are between infrared and x-ray regions. Their frequencies are between 300 MHz to 300 GHz. [22] However, for most general applications frequencies, between 915 MHz to 2.45 GHz are used. [23]

Microwaves induce two kinds of molecular motions: ionic conduction and dipole rotation. Ionic conduction is the electrophoretic movement of a molecule under an applied electromagnetic field. If the solution offers resistance to this flow of ions, the solution is heated due to the friction generated between the molecular movement and the surrounding solvent. Dipole rotation is the realignment of the dipoles in the applied field. At 2450 MHz the dipoles align and randomize at 4.9×10^9 times per second, which causes friction between the molecules and generates heat in the system. [24] [25] [23] When a sample is irradiated with microwaves, the rate of absorption of energy is dependent on its dissipation factor (tan d):

$$\tan\delta = \varepsilon'\varepsilon/$$

where e’ is dielectric loss, which is the efficiency of converting microwave energy into heat and e is dielectric constant which is the measure of the ability to absorb microwave energy. A high dissipation factor indicates less penetration of microwave energy and high absorption, which results in better heating of the samples. Table 1 illustrates dissipation factors of some of the common solvents.

[24] Due to the higher tan d values, polar solvents are used more often in MAE. Nonpolar solvents like hexane and acetone are transparent to microwaves and produce no heat during MAE.

Table 1. Physical constants of common solvents used in MAE

Solvent	Dielectric constant, e	Dipole moment	Dissipation factor, tan d ($\times 10^{-4}$)
Acetone	20.7	-	-
Acetonitrile	37.5	-	-
Hexane	1.89	-	-
Ethanol	24.3	1.96	2500
Methanol	32.6	2.87	6400
Water	78.3	2.30	1570

The basic principle of extracting actives from bio-sources, using MAE, entails heating of trace amounts of water in the plants, algae, or microbes using microwaves of appropriate power and frequency. This heating results in evaporation of the water, which induces tremendous pressure on the cell wall and causes it to rupture and release its internal components. The yields of the actives can be increased if the bio-source is soaked in a solvent with high tan d values. [25]

An MAE system has four major components: A microwave generator called a magnetron, a wave guide, which is used to guide the propagating microwaves from magnetron to a microwave cavity; a third component known as the applicator, where the sample and the sample holder are placed; and a final component—the mode stirrer, which distributes the propagating waves in various directions to heat the samples. In some systems there are also turntables for homogenous heating.

MAE systems can broadly be divided into two forms; closed and open system. In a closed system, the solvent is heated above its boiling point in a closed vessel to improve the extraction efficiency. The major advantages of this technique are temperature control and high throughput; several samples can be extracted under same conditions at the same time, no loss of volatiles. Some of the drawbacks of this technique include thermal degradation of the actives at high temperature; only materials that can handle the high temperature and pressure can be used for vessel construction. In an open system, the highest temperature at which the extraction can be conducted is determined by the boiling point of the solvent used for extraction. The major advantages of this technique are that large samples can be processed in an open vessel and the instrumentation is relatively less expensive than closed systems. Some major drawbacks are less control on the temperature and larger amounts of solvents needed for high extraction efficiency. [24] [25]

c. Factors affecting efficiency of MAE

Solvent: The solvent chosen for extraction has a tremendous impact on the extraction efficiency of the molecule of interest. The chosen solvent should have optimal solubility and high selectivity for the active under the extraction conditions. The solvent should also exhibit high dissipation factor (tan d) when irradiated with microwaves. Nonpolar solvents like hexane and chloroform are transparent to microwaves, whereas polar solvents like methanol, water, and ethanol are excellent microwave-absorbing solvents. However, mixing hexane with acetone can result in microwave heating that can extract target analytes. [26]

Temperature: Temperature is also an important factor that dictates the solubility and selectivity of a target analyte in the solvent. The ability of a solvent to solubilize a solute increases with temperature. Care should be taken in choosing temperature for thermally labile compounds. [27] Higher temperature also improves the diffusivity of the solvent in the matrix, which in turn will increase the extraction yields.

Extraction Time: The extraction yield of the analyte can be increased with time. In general, extraction times for MAE are shorter than those for the conventional solvent extractions, which reduces the risk of degradation of the labile compounds.

Microwave Power: An optimal balance needs to be reached between the microwave power and irradiation time to prevent any loss or degradation of the compound of interest.

Matrix: The physical and chemical characteristics of the matrix also play a vital role in the extraction efficiency of the analyte. Smaller particle-size matrix will yield better extraction efficiency than the one with larger particle size. Pretreatment of the matrix can also assist in improving the efficiency of extraction. Pretreating the matrix with microwave-absorbing solvents will cause the solvents to impregnate the cells and cause heating of the solvent inside and outside of the cells when irradiated with microwaves. [28]

MAE has been used for extraction of several kinds of actives such as polyphenols, essential oils, pesticides, and organic pollutants. In most cases the biggest advantage that MAE has over conventional solvent extraction is lesser consumption of solvents and shorter extraction times. [19] [24] [29] The current trend of "Green Chemistry" has led to an increase in the use of green solvents such as water in MAE. Water at ambient conditions has low Dissipation Factor, Table 1. But when subjected to heat and pressure it can act like an "organic solvent" due to decrease in dielectric constant. [24] This behavior of water has been exploited to extract a variety of flavonoids, terpenes, and polyphenols from plants. [24]

d. Ultrasonic Assisted Extraction (UAE)

Ultrasound has been used in extraction of natural ingredients as an alternative to traditional solvent extractions. UAE provides several distinct advantages over conventional extraction techniques such as use of less solvents, faster extraction times, and higher yields. [19] In UAE ultrasound frequencies range between 20 kHz to 2 MHz; in this range ultrasound is able to produce physical and chemical effects in the medium and can facilitate extraction of actives from natural sources. [30]

Unlike electromagnetic waves, ultrasound waves need an elastic medium to travel. They travel by expansion and compression cycles through the medium. A medium, which could be the extracting solvent, consists of molecules held together by certain attractive forces. When an ultrasound wave passes through this medium it causes molecules to displace from their original position, which results in successive compression and expansion phases in the medium. During the compression phase, the molecules collide with their surrounding molecules. During the expansion phase, the molecules are pulled apart and microscopic negative pressure is generated in the medium, which results in formation of a void called a cavitation bubble. This bubble is formed from dissolved gases in the medium. Successive compression and expansion cycles cause the cavitation bubbles to grow continuously until they reach a critical size beyond which they collapse during the compression cycle. This collapse results in generation of heat and formation of a transitory "hot spot" in the medium. These "hot spots" are known to have high temperature and pressure. They are able to accelerate chemical reactivity in the medium. When the cavitation bubbles collapse on the surface of solid matter in the medium, microjets and high-energy shock waves are generated. These jets and shock waves are able to destroy the cell walls of any biological material and release their contents in the extracting medium. [30]

All ultrasonic systems are composed of a transducer that converts electrical energy into sound energy by vibrating at ultrasonic frequencies. The generated ultrasound is then irradiated by an emitter. There are two common emitters used for UAE: bath and probe. In a bath system, the bio-source is exposed to a solvent in a container and then subjected to ultrasonic waves. As the system goes through successive expansion and compression, the targeted molecules are extracted in the solvent. The obtained enriched solvent is then separated from the spent biomass by centrifugation or filtration. The separated mixture is then subjected to the appropriate downstream processing to separate the analyte from the solvent. In the probe system, ultrasonic energy is irradiated by a small surface at a tip of a probe, where the probe is immersed in the extraction system. Both setups have their pros and cons. In the bath system the generated energy attenuates over time but is easy to set up and has low implementation cost. The probe system, although considered powerful and more reproducible, can cause a rapid increase in temperature in the surrounding regions of the probe. [30]

e. Factors Affecting Efficiency of UAE

In UAE, enhancement due to the use of ultrasonic waves is attributed to several mechanisms such as cell membrane disruption, improved penetration of the solvent, enhanced swelling, and capillary effect. Factors that improve the above-mentioned effects will have an impact on the efficiency of extraction. [31]

Power and Frequency: Generally, increase in power and frequency of the ultrasound waves improves the efficiency of extraction of the target analyte. [31] But it is also known that high-powered ultrasonic waves can cause a detrimental effect on the integrity of the extract by inducing high-shear forces. [32] [33]

Shape and Size of Ultrasonic Reactors: Shape of the reaction vessel is critical in determining the efficiency of extraction during UAE. As ultrasound waves are reflected and attenuated at a solid surface it is important that the right shape and size vessel is used for extraction. In the case of a probe system, the shape and the size of the tip are important and are chosen based on the extraction system. [30]

Dissolved Gases: Cavitation bubbles are formed due to the presence of dissolved gases in the solvent, where the dissolved gases act as nuclei for new cavitation bubbles. Absence of dissolved gases would make it difficult to form cavitation bubbles. On the other hand, if too many cavitation bubbles are formed, they might grow faster and result in boiling of the solvent because they would have no time to collapse. [30]

Parameters such as solvent, temperature, time, and matrix have a similar impact as they would in conventional solvent extraction. It's the efficiency of extraction that would change with the use of ultrasound.

UAE has found application for extraction of essential proteins and bioactives from a variety of bio-sources. [34] UAE improved the extraction of carnosic acid from rosemary using ethanol as the extracting solvent. The extracting yields were comparable to that obtained from the use of ethyl acetate and butanone. [35] UAE also reduced the extraction time of anthraquinones from *Morinda citrifolia* by 75% in comparison to traditional solvent extraction. [36] UAE has also been used for extraction of carbohydrates and polysaccharides. UAE was found to improve the extractability of hemicellulose from sugar cane by the cell wall and cleaving the linkage with lignin. [37] UAE has also been used with other extraction technologies such as MAE. In this example, in which natural pigments were extracted from strawberries, the optimal extraction process involved treating the biomass with MAE followed by UAE. [38]

f. Supercritical Fluid Extraction (SCFE)

SCFE is considered to be a fast, efficient, and clean method to extract actives from bio-sources. Due to these advantages, SCFE is gaining popularity over other conventional and modern extraction technologies. It utilizes supercritical fluids, which above their critical point have both liquid and gas-like properties.

When a gas is pressurized sufficiently it converts into a liquid. On the other hand, if the gas is heated beyond a certain temperature, called critical temperature, no amount of pressurization will cause it to liquefy. The corresponding vapor pressure at the critical temperature is called critical pressure, Figure 2. The junction of the two is called critical point (CP), which is unique to a given gas/solvent, and the state of the substance in the region above the critical point is called supercritical. [39] [40] Table 2 illustrates critical properties of several common solvents. [41]

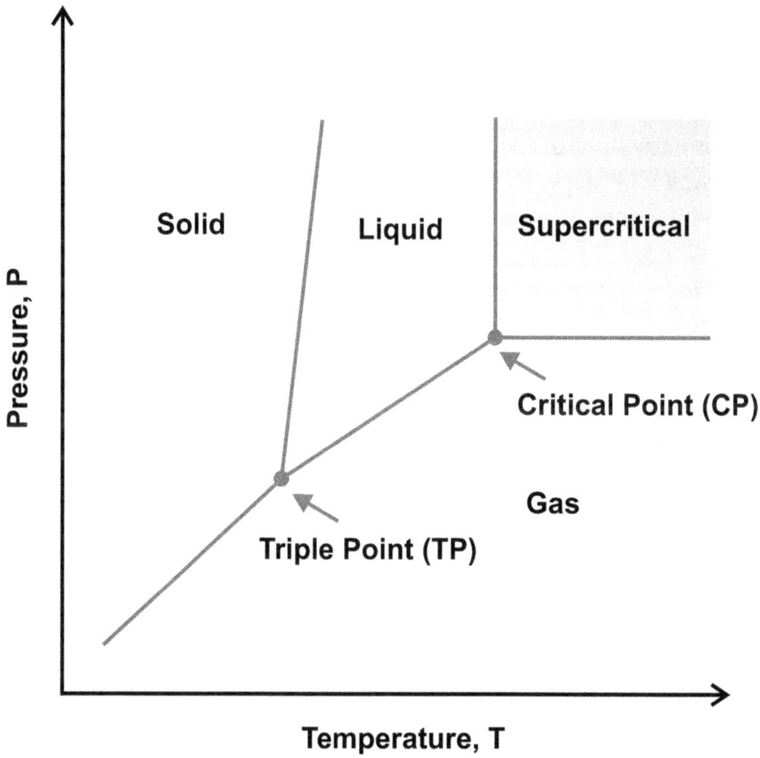

Figure 2. Pressure – Temperature diagram for a compound

Table 2. Critical properties of a few common solvents

Solvent	Critical Temperature, ˚C	Critical Pressure, MPa
Water	374.0	22.1
Methanol	–34.4	8.0
Carbon Dioxide	31.2	7.3
Ethane	32.4	4.8

This supercritical fluid has many properties of both gas and liquid. In this region minute changes in temperature and pressure can affect several solvent properties quite drastically. For extraction purposes, it can offer ideal diffusivity, viscosity, and surface tension properties. The diffusivity of this fluid is several orders of magnitude higher than the liquid solvent, which facilitates rapid mass transport. Also, low viscosity and surface tension allow for easy penetration of the biomass for extraction of actives. [41] The strong temperature and pressure dependence of solubility of active molecules in the supercritical fluid is the phenomenon that is exploited in SCFE.

The most common solvent used for SCFE is carbon dioxide; it is nonflammable, nontoxic, inexpensive, environment-friendly, inert, and nonpolluting. Processing with CO_2 results in a solvent-free extract since CO_2 is a gas under ambient conditions. Also, the critical temperature of 31.2°C for CO_2 makes it an attractive candidate for extraction of thermo-labile compounds. The efficiency of extraction of actives using CO_2 depends on the molecular weight, functional group, and polarity of the molecule of interest. In general, hydrocarbons and compounds with relatively low molecular weight can be extracted at low pressures. Nonpolar molecules with hydroxyl or carboxyl groups require moderately high pressures for their extraction. Polar compounds are poorly soluble in CO_2, and for extraction of these molecules a more polar co-solvent is often used. [40]

Figure 3 shows a schematic of a simple SCFE system. The system consists of an extraction vessel, a separation vessel, and a CO_2 source. A typical SCFE process involves the following steps: 1) extraction of the target active from the biomass; 2) separation of the active molecules from the solvent; and 3) recycling of CO_2.

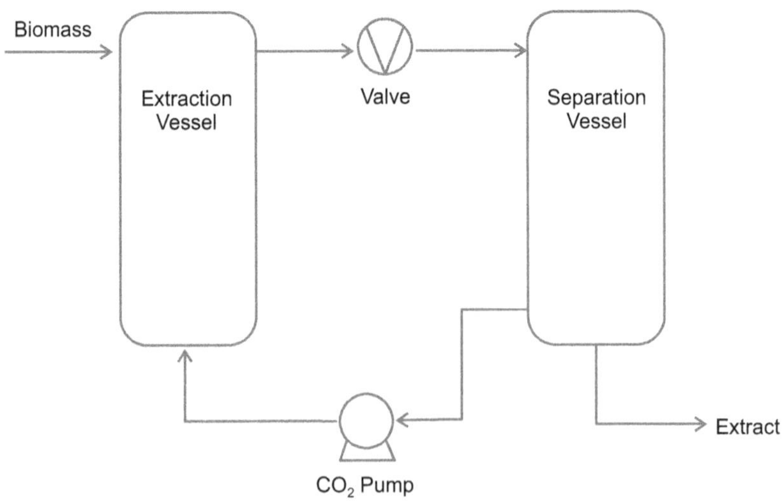

Figure 3. A schematic of SCFE – CO_2 process.

During extraction phase, the solid or liquid biomass is charged into the extraction vessel, where the biomass is then exposed to CO_2 at the desired pressure and temperature above the CP of the solvent. The target actives are extracted in the solvent phase. The resulting mixture is then sent to the separation vessel where the reduction in temperature and pressure below the CP occurs. This change causes the extracted material to precipitate. The CO_2 is then recycled to the extraction vessel where it flows through a pump that compresses the gas. The extracted material can then be further reprocessed to meet the quality parameter of the final material, which then can be used in formulations. Depending upon the complexity of the source, several modifications can be made to the process by adding multiple extraction vessels and separation vessels that can depressurize the extracted stream in a gradient that can cause selective precipitation of certain molecules based on their solubility. [40]

g. Factors affecting efficiency of SCFE

In general, parameters that improve the solubility of the active molecules in the extraction solvent tend to improve the efficiency and yield of extraction. Some of the major factors that influence the efficiency of extraction are listed below. Kinetic modeling for optimizing extraction using SCFE has also been developed by several researchers. The provided reference is an excellent review of such modeling. [42]

Biomass: It is important that the feed from which the active is to be extracted is processed optimally for extraction. Parameters like particle size, shape, porosity, and morphology play an important role. Smaller particle size provides larger surface area for the solvent matrix interaction and hence can improve the yield of extraction. But it is also important that the solids are not ground too fine because that may lead to packing of the solid material and hence channeling of the solvent. The moisture content of the biomass also plays an important role and can often compete with the extraction solvent to remove the solute from the biomass. However, in many cases removal of water to the desired level may not be possible, and in such cases other parameters would need to be optimized. [40]

Temperature and Pressure: Both temperature and pressure change the solvation power by changing the solvent density. At a constant temperature, increase in pressure results in increasing the solvent density and hence the solvating power, while at a constant pressure, increasing the temperature results in decreasing the solvent density and hence the solvation power. [39] Lower density actives such as essential oils can be extracted at low temperature and pressure. On the other hand, higher temperature and pressure are needed for extraction of larger-molecular-weight compounds such as waxes. [41]

Solvent Flow Rate: Increasing the solvent flow rate usually improves the extraction yield due to high solvent to solute ratio. This drives the solute into the solvent by keeping the solubility below the saturation limit. However in many cases it can also decrease the extraction efficiency due to reduction in contact time between the solute and the solvent. [43]

Co-Solvent: SC-CO_2 has limited ability to dissolve highly polar molecules. A co-solvent is often used to improve the polarity of SC-CO_2 for extraction of polar molecules. The choice of the co-solvent and the ratio used often depends on the active that is being extracted. Water and ethanol have been the most common co-solvents that have been used in SCFE. [44] [45] The improvement shown by the use of co-solvents can be attributed to increase in solute-co-solvent interactions and matrix swelling by the co-solvent. [40]

The versatility of the SCFE has led to it being used in many applications with a wide variety of bio-sources. For example, SCFE has been used for extraction of lipids and carotenoids from microalgae such as *Botryococcus braunii* and *Chlorella vulgaris*. [46] Essential oils have traditionally been extracted using steam distillation or hydrodistillation; however, higher temperatures used in the process can degrade the actives in the essential oil. SCFE has been used for successful recovery of variety of essential oils, without the loss in activity. [47] SCFE has also been used for extraction of natural pigments and dyes, and turmeric extract rich in curcuminoids was extracted using SCFE and ethanol as a co-solvent. The obtained extract was used as a natural yellow colorant in dairy foods. [48]

CONCLUSION

An increase in the use of natural ingredients has led to the development of several modern extraction technologies that utilize the principles of Green Chemistry. Some of the improvements achieved by these new extraction technologies are use of nontoxic solvents, use of less solvents, and generation of little to no waste from the extraction process.

In addition to the extraction method, it is equally important to choose the right source for the desired extract. Substantial variability in the amount of accumulated active(s) occurs in the plants that are harvested at different times of the year or grow in different regions. Hence it is important to obtain the biomass that exhibits little variability in target molecule(s) so that the subsequent extraction process behaves consistently. Sources that produce actives on a sub-microgram level per kilogram of the biomass will always be more expensive to extract than the source that produces them in a gram scale per kilogram of the biomass. This is true regardless of the efficiency of the extraction technology or the cost of the raw material. This can be addressed by using an optimized bio-source that hyper-accumulates the desired molecules.

The extract that is obtained by these natural processes should then be standardized so that it will behave in a consistent manner within a formulation. To achieve this, it is important to know the molecule(s) that will contribute to the efficacy of the extract. By combining the right source, optimal extraction technology and standardization, one can obtain an extract that is not only efficacious but also cost-effective, consistent, and safe.

REFERENCES

[1] F. Khachik, G. R. Beecher and N. F. Whittaker, "Separation, identification and quantification of the major carotenoid and chlorophyll constituents in extracts of several green vegetables by liquid chromatography," *J Agr Food Chem,* pp. 603-616, 1986.

[2] G. K. Jayaprakasha, L. J. Rao and K. K. Sakariah, "Antioxidant activities of curcumin, demethoxycurcumin and bisdemethoxycurcumin," *Food Chemistry,* pp. 720-724, 2006.

[3] R. F. Tayyem, D. D. Heath, W. K. Al-Delaimy and C. L. Rock, "Curcumin content of turmeric and curry powders," *Nutr Cancer,* pp. 126-131, 2006.

[4] P. B. Kaufman, L. J. Cseke, S. Warber, J. A. Duke and H. L. Brielmann, Natural products from plants, 1998.

[5] C. J. Bergman and Z. Xu, "Genotype and Environment Effects on Tocopherol, Tocotrienol, and γ-Oryzanol Contents of Southern U.S. Rice," *Cereal Chemistry,* pp. 446-449, 2003.

[6] M.-M. Oha, E. E. Carey and C. B. Rajashekar, "Environmental stresses induce health-promoting phytochemicals in lettuce," *Plant Physiology and Biochemistry,* pp. 578-583, 2009.

[7] W. A. Lotfy, K. M. Ghanem and E. R. El-Helow, "Citric acid production by a novel Aspergillus niger isolate: II. Optimization of process parameters through statistical experimental designs," *Bioresource Technology,* pp. 3470-3477, 2007.

[8] A. W. Schepers, J. Thibault and C. Lacroix, "Continuous lactic acid production in whey permeate/yeast extract medium with immobilized Lactobacillus helveticus in a two-stage process: Model and experiments," *Enzyme and Microbial Technology,* pp. 324-337, 2006.

[9] W. P. Smith, "Epidermal and dermal effects of topical lactic acid," *Journal of the American Academy of Dermatology,* pp. 388-391, 1996.

[10] N. Lourith and M. Kanlayavattanakul, "Natural surfactants used in cosmetics: glycolipids," *International Journal of Cosmetic Science,* pp. 255-261, 2009.

[11] S.-K. Kim, Marine Cosmeceuticals: Trends and Prospects, CRC Press, 2012.

[12] M. Plaza, S. Santoyo, L. Jaime, G. H. M. Garcıa-Blairsy Reina, S. F. and E. Ibanez, "Screening for bioactive compounds from algae," *J Pharm Biomed Anal,* pp. 450-455, 2010.

[13] H. Maeda, M. Hosokawa, T. Sashima, K. Funayama and K. Miyashita, "Fucoxanthin from edible seaweed, Undaria pinnatifida, shows antiobesity effect through UCP1 expression in white adipose tissues," *Biochemical and Biophysical Research Communications,* pp. 392-397, 2005.

[14] A. Pandey, D. -J. Lee, Y. Chisti and C. R. Soccol, Biofuels from Algae, Elsevier, 2014.

[15] G. Acquaah, Principles of Plant Genetics and Breeding, Wiley, 2012.

[16] D. Murphy, Plant Breeding and Biotechnology: Societal Context and the Future of Agriculture, Cambridge University Press, 2007.

[17] D. Starmans and H. Nijhuis, "Extraction of secondary metabolites from plant material: a review," *Trends Food Sci Technol,* pp. 191-197, 1996.

[18] M. D. Kostić, N. M. Joković, O. S. Stamenković, K. M. Rajković, P. S. Milić and V. B. Veljković, "The kinetics and thermodynamics of hempseed oil extraction by n-hexane," *Industrial Crops and Products,* pp. 679-686, 2014.

[19] G. Gil-Chavez, J. A. Villa, J. F. Ayala-Zavala, J. B. Heredia, D. Sepulveda, E. M. Yahia and G. A. Gonzlez-Aguilar, "Technologies for Extraction and Production of Bioactive Compounds to be Used as Nutraceuticals and Food Ingredients: An Overview," *Comprehensive Reviews in Food Science and Food Safety,* pp. 5-23, 2013.

[20] S. D. Sarker, Z. Latif and A. I. Gray, Natural Products Isolation, Humana Press, 2006.

[21] O. P. Gandhi, Microwave engineering and applications, Pergamon Press, 1981.

[22] R. Sorrentino and G. Bianchi, Microwave and RF Engineering, Johny Wiley and Sons, 2010.

[23] F. Chemat and G. Cravotto, Microwave-assisted Extraction for Bioactive Compounds: Theory and Practice, 2013: Springer.

[24] C. C. Teo, W. Chong and Y. S. Ho, "Development and application of microwave-assisted extraction technique in biological sample preparation for small molecule analysis," *Metabolomics,* pp. 1109-1128, 2013.

[25] P. Tatke and Y. Jaiswal, "An Overview of Microwave Assisted Extraction-and its Application in Herbal Drug Research," *Research Journal of Medicinal Plants,* pp. 21-31, 2011.

[26] H. Zhang, M. Xue, Y. B. Lu, Z. Y. Dai and H. H. Wang, "Microwave-assisted extraction for the simultaneous determination of Novolac glycidyl ethers, bisphenol A diglycidyl ether, and its derivatives in canned food using HPLC with fluorescence detection," *Journal of Separation Science,* pp. 235-243, 2010.

[27] K. Ganzler, A. Salgo and K. Valko, "Microwave extraction: A novel sample preparation method for chromatography," *Journal of Chromatography A,* pp. 299-306, 1986.

[28] M. Talebi, "Optimization of extraction of paclitaxel from Taxus baccata L. by use of microwave energy," *Journal of separation science,* pp. 1130-1136, 2004.

[29] V. Dragovic-Uzelac, I. E. Garofulic, M. Jukic, M. Penic and M. Dent, "The Influence of Microwave-Assisted Extraction on the Isolation of Sage {Salvia officinalis L.) Polyphenols," *Food Technology and Biotechnology,* pp. 377-383, 2012.

[30] M. A. Rostagno, J. M. Prado and G. A. Kraus, Natural Product Extraction: Principles and Applications, Royal Society of Chemistry, 2013.

[31] Y. C. Chukwumah, L. T. Walker, M. Verghese and S. Ogutu, "Effect of frequency and duration of ultrasonication on the extraction efficiency of selected isoflavones and trans-resveratrol from peanuts (Arachis hypogaea)," *Ultraso Sonochem,* pp. 293-299, 2009.

[32] L. Zhao, G. Zhao, F. Chen, Z. Wang, J. Wu and X. Hu, "Different effects of microwave and ultrasound on the stability of (all-E)-astaxanthin," *Journalof Agricultural Food Chemistry,* pp. 8346-8351, 2006.

[33] F. Kawamura, Y. Kikuchi, T. Ohira and M. Ytagai, "Accelerated solvent extraction of paclitaxel and relate compounds from the bark of Taxus cuspidate," *Journal of Natural Products,* pp. 244-247, 1999.

[34] K. Vilkhu, R. Mawson, L. Simons and D. Bates, "Applications and opportunities for ultrasound assisted extraction in the food industry — A review," *Innovative Food Science and Emerging Technologies,* pp. 161-169, 2008.

[35] S. Albu, E. Joyce, L. Paniwnyk, P. Lorimer and J. Mason, "Potential for the use of ultrasound in the extraction of antioxidants from Rosmarinus officinalis for the food and pharmaceutical industry," *Ultrasonics Sonochemistry,* pp. 261-265, 2004.

[36] S. Hemwimol, P. Pavasant and A. Shotipruk, "Ultrasonic-assisted extraction of anthraquinones from roots of Morinda citrifolia," *Ultrasonics Sonochemistry,* pp. 543-548, 2006.

[37] S. Jing, S. RunCang, S. Xiao and S. YinQuan, "Fractional and physicochemical characterization of hemicelluloses from ultrasonic irradiated sugarcane bagasse," *Carbohydrate Research,* pp. 291-300, 2004.

[38] J. Cai, X. Liu, Z. Li and C. An, "Study on extraction technology of strawberry pigments and its physicochemical properties," *Food and Fermentation Industries,* pp. 69-73, 2003.

[39] M. Mukhopadhyay, Natural Extracts Using Supercritical Carbon Dioxide, CRC, 2000.

[40] C. G. Pereira and M. A. M. Meireles, "Supercritical Fluid Extraction of Bioactive Compounds: Fundamentals, Applications and Economic Perspectives," *Food Bioprocess Technol,* pp. 340-372, 2010.

[41] A. Capuzzo, M. E. Maffei and A. Occhipinti, "Supercritical Fluid Extraction of Plant Flavors and Fragrances," *Molecules,* pp. 7194-7238, 2013.

[42] E. L. G. Oliviera, A. J. D. Silvestre and C. M. Silva, "Review of Kinetic Models for Supercritical Fluid Extraction," *Chemical Engineering Research and Design,* pp. 1104-1117, 2011.

[43] I. Papamichail, V. Louli and K. Magoulas, "Supercritical fluid extraction of celery seed oil," *Journal of Supercritical Fluids,* pp. 213-226, 2000.

[44] M. M. Barth, C. Zhou, K. M. Kute and G. A. Rosenthals, "Determination of optimum conditions for supercritical fluid extraction of carotenoids from carrot (Daucus curotu L.) Tissue," *Journal of Agricultural and Food Chemistry,* pp. 2876-2878, 1995.

[45] H. S. Park, H. J. Lee, M. H. Shin, K. W. Lee, H. Lee and Y. S. Kim, "Effects of co-solvents on the decaffeination of green tea by supercritical carbon dioxide," *Food Chemistry,* pp. 1011-1017, 2007.

[46] R. L. Mendes, J. P. Coelho, H. L. Fernandes, I. J. Marrucho, J. M. S. Cabral, J. M. Novais and A. F. Palavra, "Applications of supercritical CO2 extraction to microalgae and plants," *Journal of Chemical Technology and Biotechnology,* pp. 53-59, 1995.

[47] S. B. Glisic, D. R. Misic, M. D. Stamenic, I. T. Zizovic, R. Asanin and D. U. Skala, "Supercritical carbon dioxide extraction of carrot fruit essential oil: Chemical composition and antimicrobial activity," *Food Chemistry,* pp. 346-352, 2007.

[48] M. Braga, M. Angela and A. Meireles, "Accelerated solvent extraction and fractioned extraction to obtain the Curcuma longa volatile oil and oleoresin," *J. Food Proc. Eng,* pp. 502-521, 2007.

www.ingramcontent.com/pod-product-compliance
Lightning Source LLC
LaVergne TN
LVHW021109300926
849160LV00009B/659